Occupational Therapy Fieldwork Guide

A Student Planner

3RD EDITION

Bonnie Napier, EdD, MRA, OTR-retired,
and Jami E. Flick, PhD, OTR/L

AOTA American Occupational Therapy Association

AOTA Vision 2030
Enriching life for ALL individuals and society through meaningful engagement in everyday activities.

Mission Statement
The American Occupational Therapy Association advances occupational therapy practice, education, and research through standard setting and advocacy on behalf of its members, the profession, and the public.

AOTA Staff
Katie Jordan, *Chief Executive Officer*
Neil Harvison, *Chief Knowledge Officer*
Laura Collins, *Director of Publications*
Suzanne Takeuchi, *Vice President, Marketing and Communications*
Rebecca Rutberg, *Director, Marketing*

American Occupational Therapy Association
7501 Wisconsin Ave., Suite 510E
Bethesda, MD 20814-6519
www.aota.org

Disclaimers
This publication is designed to provide accurate and authoritative information in regard to the subject matter covered. It is sold or distributed with the understanding that the publisher is not engaged in rendering legal, accounting, or other professional service. If legal advice or other expert assistance is required, the services of a competent professional person should be sought.
—From the Declaration of Principles jointly adopted by the American Bar Association and a Committee of Publishers and Associations

It is the objective of the American Occupational Therapy Association to be a forum for free expression and interchange of ideas. The opinions expressed by the contributors to this work are their own and not necessarily those of the American Occupational Therapy Association.

ISBN: 978-1-56900-643-6
eBook ISBN: 978-1-56900-644-3
Library of Congress Control Number: 2025940861

Cover design by Steven Parrish, ESSP Design, Rockville, MD
Composition by Manila Typesetting Company, Manila, Philippines
Printed by Gasch Printing, Odenton, MD

Contents

Exercises

About the Authors

Bonnie Napier, EdD, MRA, OTR-retired, has a Bachelor of Science degree in occupational therapy from the University of Puget Sound; a Bachelor of Arts in Sociology from California State Polytechnic University, Humboldt; a Master of Rehabilitation Administration degree from the University of San Francisco; and a Doctorate of Educational Technology from Pepperdine University. She has more than 40 years of experience as an occupational therapist in clinics, hospital middle management, and occupational therapy education for occupational therapy assistants and graduate education for occupational therapists and physical therapists.

Dr. Napier "mostly" retired from occupational therapy education in 2009 after teaching in graduate programs at Dominican University of California and Samuel Merritt University, and in occupational therapy assistant programs at Yakima Valley Community College and Sacramento City College. While a doctoral student, she served as affiliated core faculty of the Stanford Geriatric Education Center, a program of Stanford University School of Medicine.

Dr. Napier's research interests have focused on cultural diversity issues in providing Western medical services, provider–client health care communication issues, and health and healing issues related to cultural beliefs. She was the first program director and fieldwork coordinator for the occupational therapy assistant program (associate of science degree) at Sacramento City College. She helped develop the curriculum and was the first academic fieldwork coordinator for the occupational therapy program at Samuel Merritt University.

This book is the result of working with hundreds of students making the transition from academic settings to the client-centered practice of occupational therapy. She now volunteers in a retirement community by teaching computer, smart pad, and computer–phone skills.

Jami E. Flick, PhD, OTR/L (she/her/ella), received her Master of Science in occupational therapy from the University of South Alabama in 2007 and doctor of philosophy in health science at Nova Southeastern University with an emphasis in global health in 2022. She joined the Pacific Northwest University of Health Sciences, School of Occupational Therapy as an associate professor and director of clinical education in September 2021.

Prior academic positions included academic fieldwork coordinator and assistant professor at the University of Tennessee Health Science Center in Memphis (2013–2021). She helped establish the Tennessee Fieldwork Consortium and served as chair from 2019–2021 to foster collaboration and support among fieldwork coordinators in the state. Internationally, Dr. Flick served as a clinical education developer and member of the Academic Advisory Committee for the first-ever bachelor's degree level occupational therapy and physical therapy program in Haiti offered by La Faculté des Sciences de Réhabilitation de Léogâne (2014–2020).

Dr. Flick has been a clinician since 2008 working across the life course in community mental health; pediatrics; inpatient and outpatient rehabilitation; and acute care, including the burn unit, trauma center, and neonatal intensive care unit. She volunteered as an occupational therapist in the Dominican Republic and Haiti. She is certified as an AOTA Fieldwork Educator, Level I Provider Sequential–Oral-Sensory Feeding Approach, Nurturing Parenting Program trainer, DIRFloortime® provider, Therapeutic Listening provider, Unyte Safe and Sound Protocol provider, facilitator for Community Action Poverty Simulations, and Mental Health First Aid. Her qualitative dissertation focused on lived experience experts in the anti-trafficking movement. She has authored book chapters on emotional regulation, health promotion, population health, and trauma-informed care.

During her "downtime," Dr. Flick enjoys brewing beer; hiking; fishing; thrift store shopping; reading; and spending time with her rescued fur babies and partner in life, Alan Jackson (not the country singer).

Preface

Level II fieldwork is an exciting, challenging time for occupational therapy students. The transition from academic work to a clinical focus brings tremendous opportunity for learning and growth. The *Occupational Therapy Fieldwork Survival Guide* is designed to prepare fieldwork students to make the most of their experience—from getting organized to working well under supervision to dealing with challenging clients. Developed from decades of experience in assisting and supervising students during their fieldwork experience, this text aims to help students not just survive but thrive as they make the transition from student to qualified practitioner.

Designed as a handbook–planner, students can use this text to self-organize for their Level II fieldwork. It is also created to be an interactive and self-reflective resource, providing space for students to

- keep track of schedules;
- note meetings and must-dos;
- organize questions to ask supervisors;
- record supervisor suggestions and comments;
- record each fieldwork site's important information;
- write goals, action plans, and timelines for completion; and
- have a record of progress from student toward entry-level practitioner!

Thoughtful exercises throughout the text guide students to thoroughly prepare for fieldwork, reflect on strengths and challenges as they engage in their new setting, and broaden their thinking with hypothetical scenarios. In addition, "Talk It Over With Your Supervisor" sections provide useful questions for students to discuss with their clinical supervisors. This new edition includes increased focus on the supervisory relationship, professionalism, and self-care. In addition, content has been revised and updated to reflect modern clinical environments.

We hope this handbook–planner contributes to your success as a fieldwork student as an occupational therapy practitioner.

To fieldwork educators: We hope this book enables students to use their short time with you effectively and will allow you to make the most of your busy schedules.

To other academic and clinical faculty: We hope this book makes a difference as you help students learn and develop into occupational therapy practitioners who make a difference, improving clients' lives.

PART I.

Personal Success Strategies

Chapter 1

Making the Transition From Student to Clinician: Preparing for Fieldwork

TOPICS

- Congratulations
- Ready?
- About your academic education
- Preparing your tool kit
- Your academic work as part of your tool kit
- Every fieldwork site is unique
- What do you need to take with you?
- Prepare for your setting
- Organizing your clinical passport: Having your compliance documents in order

After the sinking feeling that I might not be prepared for the clinic, I realized at the end of [Level I] fieldwork that I was absolutely as prepared as anything academic can prepare you for "doing." I wanted to know it all when I graduated. I came to realize that clinical practice must be lifelong learning. That you [faculty] had to teach us how to learn, not just data or specific facts. You told us there was no "absolute" approach to treatment, because IT ALL DEPENDS. I get it now: Each person, their culture, their disability, and their community create potential treatment differences. I finally get it.

—MICHAEL, occupational therapist

Congratulations

You are still a student, but your learning will continue outside the classroom. Now, your primary goal is to learn and practice occupational therapy evaluation and treatment, organize your personal needs and the needs of your clients, and work with role models who will enable you to become the best possible occupational therapy practitioner.

Just as every setting is unique, so is every student. This book has been designed to help you, the student, become your own best resource and make the most of your fieldwork experiences. You will complete your Level I experience during your academic preparation with faculty and clinical mentors providing close supervision. In Level II, you will continue to have supervision but will be expected to be more independent and provide hands-on client treatment. It's best to treat the supervisory relationship as a two-way street: You maximize your learning and grow into an independent practitioner while your fieldwork educator ensures you practice legally and ethically under their license.

This book is different from a typical textbook: It is a planner, organizer, and journal. It can provide you with a way to collect information and record your own progress. When you evaluate a client, you establish a baseline from which treatment begins. This baseline helps the client see how they change and improve. It also tells you and the third-party payers about the progress that the client is making. Good baseline information yields three results:

1. The client is more motivated when they can see quantified results.
2. You can quantify your success with the client.
3. The third-party payers are more willing to pay.

You likely will not notice your progress in becoming a clinician. Journaling what you do and how you understand what you are doing will provide your own baseline by which to measure your growth as you move from student to clinical practitioner. You will benefit from self-evaluation during this time of enormous and wonderful growth. You will soon complete your clinical education, sit for the National Board for Certification in Occupational Therapy (NBCOT®) exam, and begin that all-important first job as an occupational therapy practitioner. With this comes a great deal of responsibility to your future clients, to yourself for continuous self-growth, and to your profession.

By the time you complete Level I and Level II fieldwork, you may be nervous and worried about whether you will have had enough exposure to practice settings. Fieldwork experiences vary from program to program and from site to site, but even students from programs with 200 or more hours of Level I fieldwork experience, or three versus two Level II fieldwork placements, may still feel unsure of themselves. This uncertainty is part of your transition and is a natural feeling. This book is designed to help you increase your confidence, acknowledge and work on challenging areas, and organize your work and personal needs to maximize your learning during fieldwork.

Ready?

Here is how we envision this book helping you. Each chapter focuses on practical topics and techniques to help you better understand yourself, use resources, recognize when to consult your supervisor and other clinicians, and balance your life inside and outside fieldwork. Some of the information will be new, and some will be recommendations for organizing your work, time, and focus. The key to success in your fieldwork is learning to organize yourself and your techniques to concentrate on the clients, not your grades. You may still receive a grade for fieldwork, but the focus is on appropriate interventions and interactions with clients and coworkers. You will apply the knowledge and skills learned in the classroom. The good news is that the only examination you have left after your Level II experience is the certification examination. Your challenge then will be ensuring your actions make a difference in real people's lives.

Fieldwork is all about you and your clients' lives. In the practice setting, you cannot study all night to "ace" the exam. Your clients won't care if you were an A student or if you just squeezed by; either way, you can be a great clinician in practice. Remember that master clinicians come from all grade ranges!

You probably feel nervous and excited about starting your fieldwork. Remember that these feelings are normal. You will likely feel nervous beginning *any* new job, and your fieldwork experiences are your first jobs! Fieldwork rotations are your culminating educational courses to complete your occupational therapy education. Accountability and individual responsibility are a part of the job. You have the same responsibility to clients and coworkers that any employee would have. If you fail to provide a client with appropriate treatment, demonstrate inappropriate conduct toward a coworker, or have poor work habits, the consequences are the same as with any job but with potentially more serious effects on your career objectives and other people's lives. This book is about helping you become organized and prepared. During your fieldwork, you will learn by maintaining your focus, building good clinical organization skills, and developing professional habits that will make you the best clinician you can be. Make the most of this learning opportunity.

> *The commute to my fieldwork site was killing me, but I couldn't afford to move just for 3 months. I was driving 1 to 2 hours each way and always felt exhausted. My academic fieldwork coordinator suggested I ask around to see if someone could let me stay a couple nights a week closer to the site but NOT with occupational therapy staff because that would mix too many responsibilities during fieldwork. When I discussed this with my clinical fieldwork supervisor, he realized what a problem this had become and helped me. My work and therapy sessions improved dramatically when I solved this problem. I don't know if I would have passed this wonderful experience if I hadn't spoken up.*
>
> —SUZANNE, occupational therapy student
> at her first Level II fieldwork site

> *I was juggling child care for my 4-year-old when I started fieldwork. I was feeling guilty for not spending more time with her when I was taking classes. I had to get organized before I started fieldwork. I'd had problems that had made me late for classes, and believe me, my professors finally got through to me that this could cause even greater problems when I got to the clinic if I didn't take care of it proactively.*
>
> —SHERI, occupational therapy student

> *Even just learning to organize my clothes and lunch before I went to bed at night really helped me feel more organized and less rushed during the day. This really cut down on my feeling unorganized when I got to the clinic.*
>
> —LORI, occupational therapy student

About Your Academic Education

Like many occupational therapists or occupational therapy assistants, you may look back over your occupational therapy courses and not recall some of the content. That happens, although it is helpful to review all your course objectives and materials. Your education has been woven together with common threads, and each course has been designed to build on previous courses.

Your assignments and textbooks were chosen to help you learn and to be used as resources for your clinical work in fieldwork and beyond. Your textbooks also were selected so that during your education, you could build a personal library and have high-quality resources to use in your clinical practice. Your assignments were meant to not only test your skills and knowledge but also build examples for you to refer to in the future.

Preparing Your Tool Kit

For several years, you have focused on knowledge and skills so that you can become an occupational therapist or occupational therapy assistant. Take some time to inventory and review what you have learned. Some of the exercises in this book are designed to help you take that inventory, appreciate what you have, and identify your strengths and weaknesses. You need to accurately and honestly critique deficiencies.

You have learned a lot in school, and you have developed some distinctive skills. They may not feel unique at this moment but remember that you have been surrounded by people learning the same skills throughout the program. Occupational therapy is a special, holistic blend of anatomy, psychology, sociology, and cultural contexts that make each client an individual.

Your Academic Work as Part of Your Tool Kit

Consider the knowledge areas discussed in the *Occupational Therapy Practice Framework: Domain and Process* by the American Occupational Therapy Association (AOTA; 2020). To gauge your current understanding, review the syllabi from your courses and look through your textbooks or eBooks to review what you outlined when you took those courses. Organize your review. Using the forms in this chapter, list and check off each item, which helps you know you're accomplishing it! Your knowledge is your best pre-fieldwork tool kit. Use the exercises in this chapter and organize the tools acquired during your academic work. You'll see this statement a lot in this book: *Organize your work.*

- If you haven't done so already, organize your textbooks and eBooks by topic. If you rented eBooks or textbooks for one course at a time, consider renting additional ones that correlate with your Level II fieldwork placement so you can study for the rotation and the NBCOT exam in the future.
- Your electronic documents also should be organized. Some electronic resources let you add searchable words within the text or file name to make them easier to search and find. Create topic- or population-specific digital folders so it's easier to locate information. For example, create a folder for adult neurological conditions and add any handouts, PowerPoints, or resource sheets to that folder so you can quickly locate information about traumatic brain injuries (TBIs) during your inpatient rehabilitation rotation.
- Organize your notebooks, handouts, and syllabi—on a shelf, in a pile, or electronically. Keep the syllabi for all of your courses. You never know where you may practice in the future; some countries may require copies of your syllabi to verify your occupational therapy education and training for licensure.
- Think about the coursework you have completed while your hands work the materials. Just going through this process begins your review. When I did this, it really hit home: That difficult book from my first basic anatomy and physiology class looked a lot less imposing at the end. I really had learned something. More than 30 years later, I (Bonnie) still have that book to remind me how much I have learned and how far I have come.
- Review the way you organized information for the courses you found difficult. What helped? Being able to tell your fieldwork supervisor what helps you get organized and work most efficiently may make a huge difference in your relationship with them. Consider these questions:
    - Do you like checklists?
    - Do you recopy notes or outline readings?
    - Do you like making quick reference sheets by condensing information to one document?
    - Do you like listening or watching recordings to refresh and digest the information?
    - What works for your learning style?

Before starting Level II fieldwork, take the time to organize the valuable information and resources you obtained during your coursework (i.e., lecture handouts, assignments like group protocols and SOAP note templates). Part of this organizational process involves an actual review of materials to help you see what you already have in your tool kit and to help you appreciate that you know more than you may have realized. Stress can make you temporarily forget what you thought you knew. Preparation and organization can reduce stress, helping you become comfortable with what you know or helping you find the answers and resources for what you do not know. Remember that information changes quickly; thus, it can be more important to know where to find information quickly than to have it memorized.

Now that you have started the organizational process, complete Exercise 1.1 to explore your organizational style.

Exercise 1.1. **Organizational Reflection**

What helped you organize information in your courses? What strategies worked? For example, did you retrieve everything you needed from the learning management system (e.g., Canvas®, Blackboard®), or did you miss information? What didn't work? For example, did your file labels make it easy to identify the resource or harder? Write it down; this makes it more concrete. These organizational skills are part of your tool kit, too!

The checklist in Exercise 1.2 is one way to organize your review. Put a check mark beside each item as you complete your review. You can then visually see how your review is progressing.

Exercise 1.2. **Building the Bridge From Coursework to Fieldwork**

Add a Check Mark When Reviewed	Topic	Your Personal Feelings of Competency	Sources Reviewed That May Help You During Fieldwork (Include Books, Notes, Page Numbers, Digital Folder Name)
	Areas of occupation, activity, life roles, values		
	Occupational analysis; activity analysis		
	Matching occupation and activities to client needs		
	Cultural responsiveness and activity choices		
	Conditions, diagnoses, or referral purposes		
	Performance patterns and skills		
	Screening, assessments, and evaluation		
	Developing a plan of care		
	Designing treatment sessions		
	Documenting service delivery		

We gave you a few content areas to consider for your fieldwork preparation in Exercise 1.2. Now, use Exercise 1.3 to customize your own preparation list for your upcoming fieldwork placements. Figure 1.1 offers a different way to look at organizing your knowledge and what you have been studying to develop clinical reasoning.

Exercise 1.3. **Build Your Own Bridge From Coursework to Fieldwork**

Add a Check Mark When Reviewed	Topic	Your Personal Feelings of Competency	What Sources Did You Review That May Help You in the Clinic? (Include Books, Notes, Page Numbers, Digital Folders)

Every Fieldwork Site Is Unique

Every organization has unique qualities. Almost every clinical site is a potential fieldwork site. So, why aren't all sites good options for fieldwork? Sometimes clients with complicated needs require practitioners experienced in treating complex clients. Sometimes the supervising therapist decides whether a site has mentors available. Just because a practitioner is great with clients does not mean they will be patient with students. It is a professional responsibility to pass on information and, over time, to become a mentor, but let's face it: Not everyone is cut out to mentor.

Before you arrive at your fieldwork site, what must you know about your school and that site? What information will be useful throughout your fieldwork experience? Exhibits 1.1 and 1.2 are samples of the types of information to collect. You can organize the information about each site on the calendar pages in Part V of this book.

Exhibits 1.1 and 1.2 have blank spaces to complete before the first day at a fieldwork site. Some information can be obtained from the school's profile or from data sheets about the sites. Use your resources first. This kind of preparation is good practice for job interviews. Get the rest of the information from the site but only after you have used your resources. Your preparation saves everyone time and demonstrates your resourcefulness, which gives a favorable first impression.

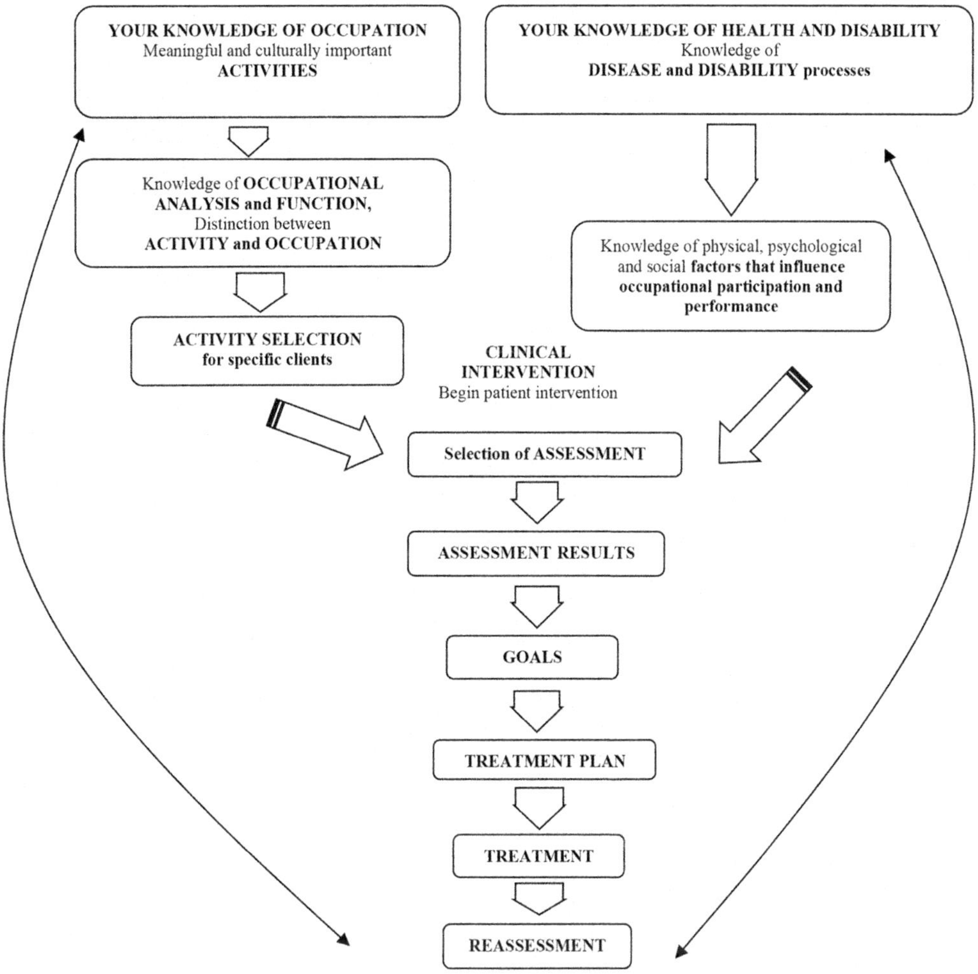

FIGURE 1.1. Activities, health and disease, and clinical intervention.

EXHIBIT 1.1. About Your School and Contacts

Your academic fieldwork supervisor's or the name of the person at the school with whom you will keep in contact: ____________________

Direct phone number for this person: ____________________

Email for this person: ____________________

Phone number to the school's occupational therapy department: ____________________

If you are injured while on fieldwork, who is your emergency contact person? Remember that if injured, you must report the injury within 24 to 48 hours.

Phone number for emergency contact: ____________________

EXHIBIT 1.2. About Your Fieldwork Sites

Dates when you are scheduled for fieldwork:

Fieldwork I Locations	Start Date and Time	Last Day
Fieldwork II Locations	**Start Date and Time**	**Last Day**

What Do You Need to Take With You?

You may do your fieldwork while living in the same location where you went to school, or you may move to a new, but less familiar, geographic area. In either case, plan ahead to know what you need to bring with you and have available during fieldwork. Take the time to organize a small space at home just for fieldwork materials and designate a space that was used for studying to organizing your client and facility information. You still will need to study, but you will be studying relevant information for delivering care to your clients, including purpose for referral, diagnoses, goals, and interventions. This defined physical space is important whether you are planning to go across the country or just a few miles away in a familiar town.

Prepare for Your Setting

Some fieldwork educators will require you to review setting- or population-specific information. Consider the primary diagnoses or reasons for referral to the sites where you will do your fieldwork. How do common conditions affect a person's occupational performance and participation? What functional limitations might they experience? Studying the common conditions you expect to see will help you recognize the functional, occupational areas that you will be assessing or treating. Formulate a list of possible problems, both common and less common. List common occupational challenges connected with the diagnoses, list common assessments that might be used, and consider what kinds of goals might be considered for the clients. Include books, websites, or other resources for the treatment commonly used by occupational therapy practitioners. These will become your information sources and justifications for the types of interventions you choose for clients.

By organizing your information, you can locate it later when your fieldwork supervisors ask you, “Why did you choose that?” or “Why did you do that?” or “What made you think that would work?” Such questions are not challenges to what you are doing. Instead, they are opportunities for you to describe your clinical reasoning, which will help you with intervention choices and explanations to fieldwork educators, clients, and family members observing therapy.

The following is a list of possible settings and diagnoses that you might encounter. This list is to get you thinking about clinical reasoning and is not intended to be a complete list of settings or potential conditions that clients may have:

- **Inpatient and outpatient rehabilitation:** cerebral vascular accidents (or stroke), TBIs, spinal cord injuries (understand level of injury), amputations, knee replacements, hip replacements, peripheral nerve injuries, and burns
- **Hand clinic:** peripheral nerve injuries, shoulder injuries, joint replacements, arthritis, cumulative trauma, carpel tunnel syndrome, and tendon injuries
- **Pediatric outpatient:** cerebral palsy, prematurity, intellectual disabilities, attention deficit disorder, hyperactivity, spina bifida, and sensory processing disorders
- **Inpatient and outpatient mental health:** bipolar disorder, schizophrenia, substance use, anxiety, and depression
- **Community-based program:** likely to be based on occupational challenges rather than diagnoses and may cover the full range of occupational dysfunctions.

For more information on common and emerging practice areas, see AOTA’s practice settings webpage: https://www.aota.org/practice/practice-settings

> *I just feel better knowing the basic questions to ask when I first get started. Let’s face it: If I don’t know what time to arrive, or where to park my car, or where the bathrooms are, or who I should be looking for, I’m going to be anxious about everything. It’s not somebody else’s responsibility to make sure things that make me nervous are covered. It’s MY responsibility! But first I have to know myself enough to know my list of questions. Even something like planning to take my lunch with me but preparing it the night before can release my anxiety about starting new things.*
>
> —CARLA, occupational therapy student planning for travel to a fieldwork site

Talk It Over With Your Fieldwork Supervisor

Prior to your arrival, ask your fieldwork educator for the most common client diagnoses and reasons for referral as well as frequently used evaluations and treatment approaches so you can familiarize yourself with information relevant for that specific site. You may be working with a more specific client population than is stated in the general information provided about the site. Ask your fieldwork educator for recommendations on resources or particular protocols that you should review, including safety and infection control protocols at your fieldwork site. You probably received training on standard precautions, such as washing your hands and wearing gloves, but ask which protocols are addressed at your site and where you can locate the supplies. Lastly, ask about basic needs, such as the fieldwork site's cell phone policies, where to park at the fieldwork site, logistics around lunch (e.g., onsite cafeteria, refrigerator or microwave available, nearby options). Ask about expectations for professional attire and limitations on artificial or long fingernails, tattoos, piercings, smoking, tobacco, and e-cigarettes.

Organizing Your Clinical Passport: Having Your Compliance Documents in Order

Every unique fieldwork site has its own process for approving a student prior to arrival. The process of sending documentation and participating in training sessions is sometimes called *onboarding*. When you go on a trip, you must organize and prepare *before* arriving at your destination. Think of onboarding to a fieldwork site like preparing for international travel. You must review the immigration rules for the country you plan to visit. You need identification documents (e.g., passport) and perhaps have to apply for travel visas or update immunizations to comply with the country's public health efforts. Similar preparation is needed for fieldwork. Most fieldwork sites require certain compliance documentation or action steps you must take in order to "onboard" you to the rotation. Your "clinical passport" provides your fieldwork site with your personal profile, immunization records, and other pertinent documentation. Most onboarding takes place electronically. Schools may use various means to help you organize your passport, including Web-based platforms like Exxat (https://exxat.com/) or E*Value by MedHub (https://www.medhub.com/software/evalue/), to store and track compliance documents. Sometimes, you may be required to upload your documents to an organization's online clinical education platform to meet their onboarding requirements. You may also have to complete applications or additional training modules that are specific to the fieldwork site to which you have been assigned.

Although your school will send your information to the fieldwork site, it's wise to carry copies (*but keep your original documents in a safe location*) on your first day to ensure the site receives your documentation on time. Usually, the site receives this information well before your arrival, but you know what? Things don't always arrive as expected. Fieldwork sites and staff change, things get misplaced or misfiled, or staff realize they needed more information for compliance. You can't start your fieldwork without completing the onboarding process to their satisfaction, so avoid potential delays. Come prepared. Be proactive. Here is the type of information typically required for onboarding:

- **Identification.** Without identification, you cannot move around your new "country"—the fieldwork site. Your school may provide an identification badge for you to wear. Your new site will likely have its own specific badges or identification, but arriving prepared with one you could use until they provide you with one shows initiative (i.e., have your school-issued badge on hand).
- **Immunizations.** Have a copy of your immunization records with you or at least up-to-date on your fieldwork management platform so you can send copies. Typically, the immunizations required by your school are adequate for onboarding to a new fieldwork site. However, be prepared that some organizations will have different requirements, especially regarding immunization exemptions. Academic programs tend to be more flexible about granting exemptions for vaccination compliance, but health care organizations may not accept exemptions granted by schools.
- **Cardiopulmonary resuscitation (CPR) certification.** Carry a copy of your current CPR certification. Most schools require students to maintain CPR certification specifically designed for health care providers that includes a hands-on checkoff for competency. Make sure you work with your academic fieldwork coordinator to ensure the certification meets the fieldwork site's standards.
- **Proof of knowledge of standard precautions and the Health Insurance Portability and Accountability Act of 1996 (HIPAA; P. L. 104-191).** Have your certificates or proof of knowledge about HIPAA and standard precautions readily available. Some organizations will require you to participate in their own training modules for HIPAA and compliance with standard precautions. This can seem repetitive or redundant, but every organization has its own process, and it is the student and school's responsibility to make sure it is followed.
- **Proof of liability insurance.** This is your malpractice insurance. You will either have purchased a policy through your school, or your school will have other arrangements for your coverage. Liability insurance is as important to you as it is to your school! Make sure you know where your copy is located for easy access.
- **Proof of health insurance.** This is an essential piece of identification at any time. Most fieldwork sites require that students show proof of personal health insurance; it is typically the responsibility of the student to maintain up-to-date coverage.
- **Accommodations for your fieldwork experience.** If you need accommodations, discuss your diverse learning needs early on with the school's disability support specialist or academic fieldwork coordinator to ensure you have the right documentation and accommodations in place before you start fieldwork. Your academic

fieldwork coordinator wants to help uphold your right to equal fieldwork education access and is there to advocate for you.

Brainstorm how personal and environmental factors may affect your performance at a fieldwork site and establish an understanding of when and how to share your need for accommodation during the process. Accommodations are not retroactive; rather, they begin only after you have provided the necessary information to determine the access needs and engage in the interactive process to make the best decisions regarding a plan of action. So, if you start fieldwork and then realize you need accommodations, there's no going back to change past fieldwork evaluations of your performance before the accommodations. Use every tool and support mechanism to your advantage.

Your academic fieldwork coordinator will have sent most of the aforementioned content to the site before your arrival. But sometimes, especially in large health care centers, complications can arise that delay your onboarding and potentially affect your start date. For example, your background check took longer than expected to process and you cannot arrive on-site until Human Resources clears it. Be proactive and work ahead to prevent delays when possible. As soon as you have access to your onboarding instructions, get started right away! Besides, it makes a good first impression if you have your clinical passport up-to-date and fully in compliance on your first day.

See Exhibit 1.3 for a checklist to ensure your documents are up to date, accessible, and safely stored.

- Take copies of the important documents to the site. *Always keep the original documents in a safe place* and carry only the copies.
- You may need to show original forms, and the site will keep a copy in their records. Keep your original documents together in one envelope or file folder.

Summary

This chapter focused on helping you prepare for the transition from a full-time student in the classroom to a student practitioner. You have determined your own way to review your materials before going to your fieldwork sites, and you may have made a list: things to help you prepare, useful content or books to review, how to dress at your particular sites (e.g., street clothes vs. laboratory coat), and what to expect. Your list may have grown after communicating with your fieldwork educator to identify key content areas to review and prepare for your first day. You also received an overview of the "clinical passport" and onboarding process that permits you entry to the fieldwork learning experience at your rotation site.

Continue to discover other ideas that will keep you proactive and help you to get the most out of your fieldwork experiences.

EXHIBIT 1.3. Onboarding Checklist

Copy Into Folder	Item	Where Is the Original?
	Identification badge (either facility or school-issued)	
	CPR for health care providers certification	
	Tuberculosis (TB) skin test results or letter confirming a TB negative chest X ray	
	Hepatitis B immunization	
	Varicella (chicken pox) immunization or proof of immunity	
	Measles, mumps, and rubella immunization and/or titer report	
	COVID-19 vaccination proof	
	Proof of liability insurance (this may be provided by the school or student)	
	Proof of health insurance	
	Proof of accommodations	
	Background checks	
	Drug screen results	
	Other specific request from fieldwork sites	
	Other specific request from fieldwork sites	

References

American Occupational Therapy Association. (2020). Occupational therapy practice framework: Domain and process (4th ed.). *American Journal of Occupational Therapy*, *74*(Suppl. 2), 7412410010. https://doi.org/10.5014/ajot.2020.74S2001

Health Insurance Portability and Accountability Act of 1996 (HIPAA), Pub. L. 104–191, 42 U.S.C. § 300gg, 29 U.S.C §§ 1181–1183, and 42 U.S.C. §§ 1320d–1320d9.

Chapter 2

Preparing for the Fieldwork Experience and Supervisory Relationship

TOPICS

- Preparation
- Developing a growth mindset and receiving feedback
- Being proactive

Preparation

Be prepared for meeting with your supervisor and working with your clients. Learn as much as you can about the fieldwork site and fieldwork educator ahead of time. Most schools have site profile information available that students can explore, including information in their fieldwork management systems or student learning platforms. You might have access to the site's past student fieldwork evaluations and other site data, such as the treatment population they serve, typical hours, and tips for preparing for the fieldwork experience. You can also perform your own online search to learn about the practice setting.

Ask questions about the site and supervisor during your introductory communication through emails, phone calls, or virtual meetings. Have a list of questions ready, but make sure you thoroughly review site profiles so you don't ask questions that are already answered in the site profile information. Exhibit 2.1 provides introductory email with sample questions.

EXHIBIT 2.1. Sample Introductory Email

Hello, Dr. or Ms. Smith (if you know the credentials),

I am Olga Thompson, a first-year Master of Science Occupational Therapy student at [School Name]. I have been assigned to [Fieldwork Site Name] for a Level I fieldwork [or Level II fieldwork] rotation during [dates]. I am excited about this opportunity and look forward to meeting you and the team. To prepare for the rotation, I'd like to verify some details:

1. Where and what time would you like me to arrive on the first day?
2. What is the dress code? [If the dress code is listed, then verify the dress code or ask questions, if needed.]
3. May I bring lunch and snacks? Will there be a place to store food and each lunch?
4. What compliance documents (if any) should I bring with me?
5. Do you have any specific things you'd like me to read or review to arrive prepared?

Sincerely,
[professional signature line with phone number and email for contact]

The fieldwork educator or site coordinator may send you resource packets and weekly objectives. If you receive suggestions for materials and content to review, or you are given access to resources, then take advantage of the opportunities and arrive prepared on your first day. Arriving without reviewing relevant material or practicing necessary skills for the practice setting can give the impression that you are not committed to the learning experience. Seize every opportunity to learn and grow!

Developing a Growth Mindset and Receiving Feedback

Fieldwork is a bridge between academia and clinical performance in which someone always provides feedback about success, grading, timelines, and performance. In the workplace, you usually get minimal feedback unless you mess up or don't get things done in a timely manner, or you learn to ask for information without sounding like you're saying, "Am I doing it right? Am I doing it right?" which can become annoying to clinicians trying to get their work done and can make you sound like you lack confidence and awareness of your strengths and weaknesses. Learning how to ask for feedback influences the value and content of the responses you will receive.

Seeking Appropriate Feedback

No needs, no referral. No referral, no services or reimbursement for those services! Face it: When you're doing a good job, *you'll be doing what is expected.* When you do something wrong or endanger clients, it is *then* that you're going to hear about it. You'll feel as though you aren't receiving much feedback about what you do well. This is a tough transition, but you're in the real world. In the real world, good work earns you a paycheck and usually a good annual review, but you immediately hear about the bad work.

This doesn't mean there's no positive feedback; it's just different from what you've received in school. Your fellow clinicians will give you positive feedback, but it's in different forms: "You've done a great job with Mr. Jones," "That was a creative intervention with Mrs. Smith," "I'm going to try that with one of my patients."

Your clients will also give you feedback. "How do you stay so patient with us?" or "Thank you for helping me," for example. And sometimes: "Just leave me alone." But other times, your peers will be too busy, and the clients may feel the pain before the gain is apparent. You need to develop confidence and seek appropriate feedback, making yourself open to constructive feedback, even if it is negative. Without feedback, you will miss great opportunities to improve.

Have you ever heard the story about a speaker with a big piece of spinach stuck in their front teeth? People didn't remember the speaker's words—just the spinach. All someone needed to do was tell the speaker, before they started talking, so the spinach could've been removed—and everyone would have focused on the words instead of the spinach. So, what's *your* "spinach"? It could be a distracting gesture. It could be touching a client before they are ready. It could be that you don't put away treatment materials and others resent cleaning up after you. Positive feedback is easy to accept. Negative feedback needs to be evaluated, and you need to make a plan for change as needed. Changing is never as easy as being congratulated on what you already do, but if you miss the opportunity, you also miss the chance to become the best possible clinician!

Dealing With Negative Feedback

Dealing with positive feedback is easy. Handling negative feedback or constructive criticism can be harder. Dweck (2016) coined the term *growth mindset* (vs. a *fixed mindset*) to describe a mental state that helps with success. With a growth mindset, you believe that you will be more successful by working hard, developing productive strategies, and incorporating input from others into your practice. A fixed mindset reflects the belief that your talents are innate and cannot be honed. In general, people who worry less about looking smart and instead devote their energy to growing and learning (i.e., growth mindset) are more successful.

How do you react to negative criticism? You can choose how to deal with it. Consider the suggestions in Figure 2.1 for dealing with criticism and leveraging a growth mindset. Where do you stand? You can't change what you won't admit needs changing, and you can't learn if you can't see where the gaps exist in your own knowledge.

Have you ever said, "I don't even know what *questions* to ask." That is the first step in critical self-appraisal, but you must move from that point to embrace a willingness to ask others where to begin or how to clarify your questions. Once you know the questions, search your tool kit for answers, or ask others about tools to add to your tool kit. That's the positive approach to negative feedback. Recognize the opportunity for growth.

Evaluating Yourself

How skilled are you in accepting feedback? The grid in Exercise 2.1 can help you recognize how you usually respond. Where you are in accepting feedback will vary. Some people make it easier than others to take their feedback, but you always have a choice of how to receive it. Do some people make you feel more defensive? Your defensiveness may interfere with hearing what is really being said, causing you to miss

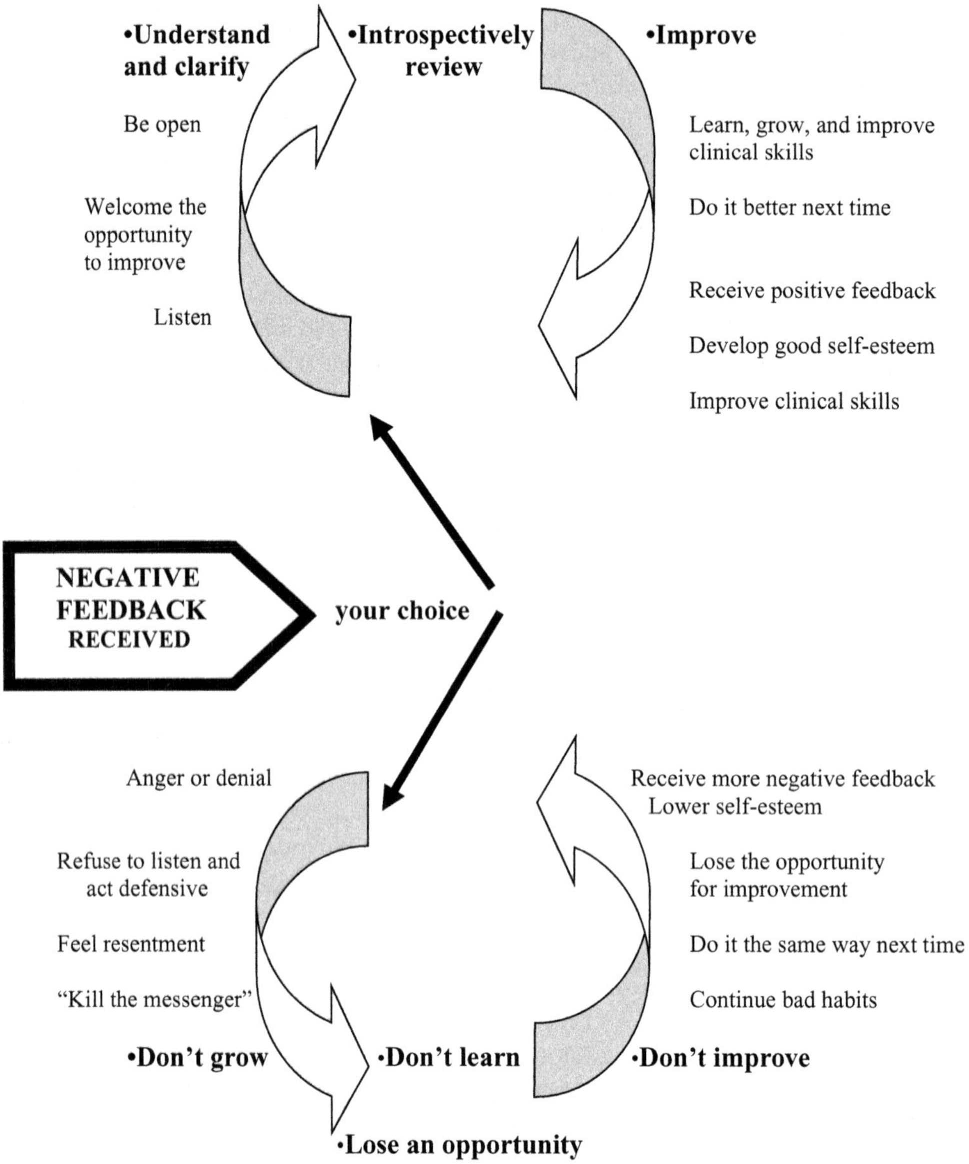

FIGURE 2.1. Dealing with negative feedback.

an opportunity to improve. Busy people can be brisk and abrupt. This doesn't mean that you should disregard their feedback. It also doesn't mean that they don't like you or are judging you. It just means they are busy, and their abruptness may have nothing to do with you. Remember that you are moving from focusing on academic progress to concentrating on your client's progress.

Exercise 2.1. How Do I Respond to Feedback?

Evaluate your response to feedback (see Figure 2.1). On the lines below, state the problem or issue about which you are concerned and describe it as concretely as you can. Putting thoughts in writing can be a powerful way to be introspective and clarify what you want to communicate.

____

____

____

____

____

Then, using the grid that follows, indicate how positively you see yourself at this moment for each item listed.

Where Do You See Yourself Today?

Positive	++	+	?	–	– –	Negative
Actively listen						Am defensive, ignore
Envision or create opportunity, be open						Am resentful
Understand and clarify						Don't listen, don't grow
Engage in introspective review						Ignore feedback
Do it better next time						Do it the same again and again
Have good self-esteem, see growth toward becoming clinician						Have poor self-esteem, ignore a chance to grow

Note. ++ = very positive; + = positive; ? = unsure; – = negative; – – = very negative.

Next, answer the following eight questions:

1. What can I do to change how I view and communicate the problem?

____

____

____

____

2. Do I need to listen more carefully to the content rather than react to the tone? What might I be ignoring?

____

____

3. Is this an opportunity for me to change and become a better clinician?

4. What can I do to deal effectively with this situation?

5. If I need to confront someone, how can I phrase it so that I do not increase my own or the other person's defensiveness? *Write out variations of what may be said.*

6. How could I review the situation and avoid being hypersensitive about comments that could have a different meaning than what I thought I understood?

7. Have I asked a significant, unbiased person (e.g., not my best friend who always agrees with me) about other ways to interpret the situation?

8. After dealing with the situation, what were the best approaches I used and why? What are the approaches I should avoid, and why?

Best approaches	**Why are these "best approaches"?**
Approaches I should avoid:	**Why should I avoid these approaches?**

Talk It Over With Your Fieldwork Educator

Ask your fieldwork educator what kind of formal and informal feedback you can expect to receive at your fieldwork site. Sometimes it helps to know ahead of time. Most of us occasionally sound or appear to be abrupt. Listen to the words, not the tone. Be aware of your own words and tone.

I had a lot of trouble with one therapist where I was doing my Level II fieldwork. She had given me a patient of hers, a boy with muscular dystrophy. His usual treatment had been to follow her around the pool so he got some exercise. He usually started complaining before the first lap around the pool was completed and asked, "Can I get out?" "Could we stop?" or "Why do I have to keep going?" I changed what we were doing in the pool. We began playing pool basketball. I'd move the floating basket to keep him moving and often throw the ball over his head or to a different corner of the pool so he kept moving. It was the same movement and incorporated his upper extremities more than walking laps in the pool.

The therapist complained to my clinical supervisor that I was making therapy too much fun and that his parents might see it as play rather than work. The boy began asking to stay longer in the pool exercising with basketball. The therapist insisted that I be reprimanded. After thinking over the negative feedback, I asked my clinical supervisor to observe my treatment session. I thought it was positive that I made it more fun for the patient, and while I might not be able to count laps, I could quantify the amount of time he kept moving at a good pace. The other therapist wouldn't budge on her opinion. Our compromise was that I would gradually change him back to walking laps in the pool to make the change back to his original therapist easier when I completed my fieldwork. I still think it is better to make therapy (and learning) more fun!

—BONNIE, occupational therapist (and co-author of this book), on my fieldwork experience

When receiving feedback, a good introspective review will tell you which of the following actions you need to take:

- **Change.** Evaluate other ways to do the action or activity that brought criticism and provide a better explanation. Explain *why* you are doing or should not be doing the suggested correction, and always be prepared to answer, "Why are you doing that?" regardless of the person's tone of voice. If you cannot provide a reason why, you should not be doing it, or you may not understand all the implications your supervisor wants you to consider.
- **Ignore the feedback.** Not all feedback needs action, but this should be your last choice, only if your self-assessment supports it. Be prepared to explain why you ignored the input.

Understand that anger and resentment are cues that you are not listening.

Use Exercise 2.1 to evaluate concretely how you are doing when you receive difficult feedback. In Chapters 15 and 16, you can find additional copies of this exercise, which you can use to help you assess what is happening when you receive difficult feedback and to keep track of feedback, reactions, and progress. You may see patterns in your problems and your successes. If you can change the way you receive feedback, it may provide you with a great opportunity for growth.

Being Proactive

One of the best ways to decrease your stress and thereby increase your flexibility and ability to communicate and negotiate is to be proactive. Being *proactive* means that you plan ahead and consider possible consequences. Doing so enables you to consider a variety of options from which to choose. You focus on selecting the desired outcome. You become aware of how your choices along the way lead to the results. You practice *STP*: *S*top, *t*hink, and *p*lan before acting.

Being *reactive* means waiting until a situation occurs before responding to it. You may be caught by surprise and then respond impulsively. You don't have time to consider the options and may choose a short-term solution that results in a long-term problem for you and your client.

Think It Through

Preparation for working with clients is essential. Let's look at this example: You know you need to transfer a client from bed to wheelchair, and you have not seen this client before. In one scenario, if you go into their room unprepared, you are setting the stage for reactive actions. One consequence would be that you and the client end up on the floor with one or both of you injured. In real-life situations like this, lack of planning has resulted in broken bones, concussions, and injured backs for clients and practitioners. In a different scenario, say the client is in a residential mental health facility because of a new onset of psychosis and concerns the client could be a threat to themself or others. If you go into their room unprepared, you might not be ready to minimize risk and could harm the client or yourself.

Okay, that gives you some idea about possible consequences. What can you do to be proactive? Exhibit 2.2 offers factors to consider and actions to take when transferring a client you have not seen before.

Plenty of unexpected things happen in everyone's lives or daily activities. If you plan for those things that can be anticipated, you will have more time to focus on those things that cannot. A proactive person does not need to experience all situations to effectively plan and prevent problems during client treatment or during interactions with coworkers.

EXHIBIT 2.2. Solving the Problem: Transferring an Unfamiliar Client

Considerations or Questions	Action
Look up the client's diagnosis or referral information.	• Find out what kinds of transfers are usually recommended with this type of client.
Review the customary transfer techniques for this type of client.	• To avoid having to say, "I guess I should have asked," ask your supervisor to go over the most commonly used transfer techniques at the site. Many rehabilitation teams have worked out preferred transfer techniques. • Review your course and lab notes. What do they say about this type of situation? Remember that even an experienced therapist who is new to a clinic has to ask these questions.
What are the precautions usually associated with this diagnosis?	• Identify whether this client is impulsive and needs cuing for safety. • Determine whether they have potential muscle tone problems that need to be assessed. • Find out if any visual problems are likely. • Review the client's medical chart to ascertain weight-bearing status.
Review the latest information in the medical chart to see how other members of the treatment team transferred the client.	• This review gives you some history; however, remember that a lot depends on the individual clinician and client.
What do you do if the client begins to slip during a transfer?	• Practice with a willing substitute. Proactive planning for the possibility of unexpectedly lowering the client to the floor is much safer for all than unexpectedly hitting the floor! You can do this! Plan accordingly for success!

Consider Your Challenges to Being Proactive

As you work with clients and develop a routine, try to identify the areas that challenge or prevent you from being proactive. For example, a creative occupational therapist found they had trouble recalling some of the treatment ideas they had considered for their clients. The therapist worked in a fast-paced environment with back-to-back clients. Treatment ideas would pop in their head after-hours; by the time they were back at work, the ideas were long gone. The therapist's solution? They made a note folder on their smartphone and added treatment ideas to it. Each folder had one client's initials on it, and when ideas came to the therapist for that client, they entered notes into that folder. The therapist would sometimes share their notes with other therapists—at first because this other therapist struggled with a client's treatment routine. Gradually, other occupational therapy practitioners and support staff adopted the note-taking idea. It became a common way to initiate sharing of treatment needs and ideas.

Critique Yourself

Make a list of things that you optimally could or should change about yourself, your habits, or your routines related to work. Be honest: You don't have to share the list with anyone else! Once you have identified the things that need to change, you may ask someone to help you change. Remember: You cannot improve if you do not know what needs changing. Developing personal insight through self-reflection and making changes where needed will help you become an effective, ever-evolving clinician. Use Exercise 2.2 to begin identifying challenges.

> *I had trouble getting documentation done quickly. I'd carry the information in a jumble in my head but would feel flustered when I tried to write—and I was normally a good writer. Documentation just seemed different. I thought carrying a notebook or a clipboard sounded like a really awkward solution, and besides, wouldn't the client think you're less attentive to them if you kept writing stuff?*
>
> *With practice, I found that the clipboard wasn't at all distracting. In fact, it made clients feel important because I was taking notes about them! In the beginning, I was forever leaving my clipboard in someone's room or setting it down and forgetting it for a few minutes. That's also when I realized it was important to use initials or some other identifier to keep client information confidential if I did leave it where it could be read by someone else. Now, my clipboard looks like a casual part of me, but it has taken practice to make it feel casual.*
>
> —ROBERTO, occupational therapy assistant student on his second Level II fieldwork assignment

Exercise 2.2. **Where Are Your Challenges?**

What creates difficulty for you? Where do your challenges lie? Managing a tight schedule or a fast pace? Organizing equipment you'll need during treatment? Getting documentation done efficiently? Write down your challenges so you can concretely think of solutions:

____

____

____

____

____

____

____

Plan Proactively for an Unfamiliar Fieldwork Site

The earlier example involving transferring an unfamiliar client illustrated how to be proactive in planning that single activity. Now consider planning for a large, personal activity, such as going to an unfamiliar clinical site. Using Exhibit 2.3, consider factors and questions as well as what actions to take in the scenario that you will be working in an unfamiliar city or location without a support network. You will need to focus on adjusting to the new fieldwork site and providing occupational therapy as quickly as possible. How can you be proactive? Then, using Exercise 2.3, develop your own proactive questions.

EXHIBIT 2.3. Solving the Problem: Working at an Unfamiliar Fieldwork Site

Considerations or Questions	Action
How do I learn about my new location?	• Search the internet for the local chamber of commerce for information on the fieldwork site. • If cell service is unreliable, as in some rural areas or in underground subways, obtain maps or travel books. You can access these resources from the American Automobile Association (commonly known as AAA), local welcome centers, or retailers and convenience stores. • Search your GPS or electronic device for maps and pin the locations you need. • Ask the fieldwork educator for tips and tricks for getting around and things to do. • Find other resources on the Web. • Practice your travel route before the first day to be sure you can arrive on time.

I'm worried about staying in touch with my support network. I'm worried about social isolation in a new place.	• With reliable cell phone service or internet access, you can set up weekly social check-ins with classmates, friends, and family—preferably with video access so that you can see their warm, welcoming faces. • If cell service or internet access serves as a barrier, consider a landline or letter-writing for distance communication. • Ask your fieldwork educator for tips on connecting with others in the area. • Consider building new social connections with those who share your interests, spiritual practices, and hobbies.
I can't afford a cell phone and some of the other expenses without working.	• If possible, before beginning at this fieldwork site, talk to your academic fieldwork coordinator about your financial barriers. Stipends or other benefits may be offered through your school to support you. • Balancing work and fieldwork is extremely difficult! You will be earning a good salary when you complete Level II fieldwork in a few months. Your student loans may be mounting, but in the long term, don't sacrifice your safety or health and don't sacrifice the learning that is possible during fieldwork for a few hundred dollars (based on my experience). You will never again have the opportunity to learn what is available to you during fieldwork! You are not paying to work for free. You are paying tuition for the intensive work that went into vetting and securing the fieldwork site and allowing for continued access to resources (e.g., library, student affairs, faculty mentors).

Exercise 2.3. Identifying Your Proactive Considerations or Questions and What Actions Need to Be Taken

Considerations or Questions	Action

Use Your Resources to Take a Proactive Approach

Being proactive does not mean asking someone what to do; it means looking for your own answers. Dobyns (2019) lists proactiveness as one of the top things you can do to master your fieldwork experience and suggests that if, for example, you "see a patient with a condition you haven't treated before, such as fragile X syndrome, research it in advance" (para. 2). First, you review your own resources and formulate possible answers. Your resources may include notes from an academic course, textbooks, reference books, the internet, or other colleagues.

After looking at your resources, consider additional questions you might ask and whom you might ask. It is better to write out your questions so you can reread them to ensure they make sense and that you include only important questions. Just as you need to consider whether resources are credible when gathering information, you must consider who will be the best person to provide information. You need to know how to formulate a clear question to get the information you seek and your resources' reliability. The two scenarios in Exercise 2.4 can help get you started on creating solutions during your fieldwork.

Exercise 2.4. **Posing Questions and Creating Solutions**

Devise a technique to pose questions to yourself and create solutions that might work well for you during fieldwork. Writing ideas down helps to clarify your thought process. Consider the following two scenarios, and think about who will get the most from the ensuing dialogue:

Scenario 1. Occupational therapy student Adrian is unsure how to work with a complex client with the initials C. X. Adrian considers two approaches but isn't sure either will work. They have weighed the pros and cons of each and written what they see as possible reasons to use either one. Adrian meets with their fieldwork educator, presents the possibilities, and demonstrates that they have thought about solutions rather than just saying that they are unsure where to begin with treatment.

Scenario 2. Harper is unsure how to work with a complex client with the initials F. Y. "Oh, well," Harper thinks, "my fieldwork supervisor will have the answer." They ask their supervisor, "What should I do with F. Y.?"

Now, suppose that neither Adrian nor Harper can interrupt the activity in which their fieldwork supervisor is involved, so they need to act on their own. Write your answers to the following questions:

1. Which student—Adrian or Harper—is most likely to work out a solution? ________________
2. Which student is most proactive? ________________
3. If the fieldwork supervisor is available to meet, which student will likely have the most productive, collegial discussion? ________________

How Proactive Are YOU?

What causes you problems when you intend to be proactive? What can you do to be the best student clinician you can be? Consider your list of challenges to being proactive (see your work in Exercise 2.2) and then complete Exercise 2.5. Refer to Exercise 2.5 when challenging scenarios emerge during your fieldwork experience and add to it, expanding as your tools for success in your tool kit. Part of being proactive is considering multiple options—not just one. Some options may seem impossible until you consider what small steps you can take to make them possible. Problem solving is a creative process.

Exercise 2.5. Being Proactive: Challenges and Techniques

Your Challenge to Being Proactive	Techniques to Increase Proactive Skills
I feel embarrassed when I ask my fieldwork educator questions. I think they think I should already know the answers and get irritated with me.	Maybe I'm feeling intimidated when that isn't at all my supervisor's intention. My educator is always in a rush in the clinic; it isn't just about me. Maybe we could work out a way in which I could leave notes with questions to answer later. Or maybe we could use email or text messaging to communicate, which would feel less intimidating to me.
List a challenge:	Devise some solutions:
List a challenge:	Devise some solutions:
List a challenge:	Devise some solutions:
I don't know what the most common problems are in the setting I'm going to.	I can formulate a question to ask about what kinds of clients are seen at the setting. That's a reasonable question to help me become familiar with a setting. I can make my own list to get the discussion going.
List a reason for referral:	List common treatments or interventions:
List a reason for referral:	List common treatments or interventions:
List a reason for referral:	List common treatments or interventions:

Flexibility

Once you are engaging in the fieldwork experience and applying your knowledge and skills, consider the multiple possibilities that you will encounter during evaluations and treatment sessions with clients. What is the best that could happen? What is the worst that could happen? And what is in between and might be good enough? This kind of thinking is a lot like planning graded activities when you were learning treatment planning: Everything has multiple possibilities. Thinking about multiple options will help stretch and flex your clinical creativity and problem-solving ability and provide you with insight into various possibilities. Further, by becoming more flexible in clinical situations, you strengthen your ability to see new options and be proactive.

Summary

Preparing for fieldwork requires more than getting organized. It also means preparing your mindset and openness to feedback, an essential part of the learning process. Preparation also involves being proactive—that is, planning ahead—so that you can avoid acting impulsively. Whether you are doing personal planning to keep yourself more focused during fieldwork or are thinking about multiple options for a client so you can respond to unexpected treatment situations, being proactive reduces stress; makes you more efficient; and allows you to consider the pros, cons, and possible issues involved in various options to ensure your interventions improve client outcomes.

Reference

Dobyns, K. (2019). *Mastering fieldwork.* https://www.aota.org/publications/student-articles/fieldwork/mastering-fieldwork

Chapter 3

Goal Setting

TOPICS

- Using values to guide goals
- Knowing your personal and professional mission statements to set measurable goals
- Evaluating goals using RUMBA
- Moving forward with your personal and professional goals
- Leveraging tools and resources for goal achievement
- Exploring habits that help, habits that hinder
- Staying motivated
- Creating client goals

When I was beginning my Level II fieldwork experience, I wrote what I considered to be a good goal for my client. My clinical fieldwork supervisor rejected it, and when I asked why, she told me that "it wasn't an appropriate goal for documentation." I still didn't get it, and my supervisor didn't seem to know how to clarify for me. The goal I had written was: "Complete patient evaluation."

For a long time, I didn't understand why my goal was unacceptable. Then it dawned on me: "Complete patient evaluation" was MY goal. It was written in terms of my behavior, not the patient's. I looked at it another way: The patient didn't care if I completed the evaluation or not; she just wanted to get better. The insurance company didn't care if I completed the evaluation; it just cared if I was able to document appropriate treatment progress. MY goal spoke only to what I needed to get done. That was when I finally separated MY goals from the patient/client-focused goals.

—ELENA, occupational therapist

Using Values to Guide Goals

Good goals are aspirations supported by our *values*, the standards determining what we believe to be most important in life. Values form the basis for our decisions and actions and lead us to perform to our best ability. Before getting down to the business of creating specific goals, take some time to think about your values. Factors that influence the development of values include family, spirituality, friends, peers, coworkers, school or education, culture, and society. As a health professional, you have at least three areas that influence your values:

- **Social values.** These values are held in common by most society or cultural group members and are considered guidelines for the "right" way to live and conduct oneself (Social Value International, n.d.). The group may be a political one, an economic one, family, extended family, or other groups that influence one's perception of the environment and interactions with others. Sometimes, this interaction is called *group pressure* (American Psychological Association, 2018).
- **Professional values.** These values are developed by and for a professional group. They form the basis for professional codes of ethics. In health care practice, values generally emphasize the need for and means of dedicating one's efforts to clients' well-being. Professional values may vary among professional organizations and the agency where one is employed, and they can differ significantly among employers (Almutairi et al., 2022; Mannion & Davies, 2018).
- **Personal values.** These values are developed independently from one's society or professional peers. Personal values sometimes differ from and conflict with social or professional values. They are a person's internally held values. Peer pressure can influence an individual's external behaviors to differ from their internally held values (Ethics Resource Center, 2014).

Values make sense of the core beliefs that guide our lives. Integrity achievement, choice of personal goals, responsibilities to others, relationships, respect, definitions of fairness, and responsibilities to others as a team member are all influenced by values. We even define *health, wellness, disability,* and *illness* relative to our beliefs and values. For example, some cultures value autonomy and accepting personal responsibility for the state of one's health. Other cultures believe that health is determined more by the will of a higher power or by fate than by the activities of the individual, and responsibility is assigned to a group—occasionally at the expense of the individual (Agency for Healthcare Research and Quality, 2024; Gurung, 2019).

Your values influence your career choice and will continue to influence your professional activities and decisions. Creating goals provides an opportunity to concretely review your values and beliefs to determine the best path forward. You may discover some long-held values are no longer aligned with your evolving professional values and that you want to change. For example, suppose you valued staying up late and sleeping in on weekends but discovered it throws off your sleep hygiene and routine, lowering your endurance for the work week. You may want to consider incorporating new values into your professional and personal goals, so you can thrive as an occupational therapy practitioner. Complete Exercises 3.1 and 3.2 to explore your values.

Exercise 3.1. Identifying Your Personal Values

What are your 10 most important values? Consider the following examples:

- **Honesty.** People can trust what I say. I admit my mistakes and take steps to correct them.
- **Fairness.** I treat others with respect and consideration. I try to understand other people's views without argument or judgment.
- **Trustworthiness.** Others can count on me to follow through on promises and commitments. They can depend on me to arrive on time, finish what I start, and complete assigned tasks.

Now, using these examples as a guide, write 10 values of your own. That may seem like a lot, but dig deep and think about what you value:

1. ____________________
2. ____________________
3. ____________________
4. ____________________
5. ____________________
6. ____________________
7. ____________________
8. ____________________
9. ____________________
10. ____________________

Talk It Over With Your Fieldwork Supervisor

Talk with your fieldwork supervisor about their values. You might ask the following questions:

- What are your opinions about professional values for occupational therapy practitioners?
- What values drive the organization of this fieldwork site?
- How are the organization's values manifested in action?
- How do you resolve conflicts among social, professional, and personal values?

Exercise 3.2. **Checking Your Values for Consistency**

Look at the values you listed in Exercise 3.1 and write each one in the first column. Indicate to what degree each is consistent with your actions. In other words, do you "walk your talk?" If not, why not? In the third column, indicate what steps you could take to change your actions to better align with your values.

Value Previously Listed	Is This Value Consistent With Your Actions?		Plan to Make This Value More Consistent With or in Alignment With Your Actions
	Yes	No	

Knowing Your Personal and Professional Mission Statements to Set Measurable Goals

A *mission statement* articulates a person's life aspirations. It is based on our personal and professional values, which are the guiding principles for our actions. This statement serves as the foundation for our goals, and each goal moves us closer to accomplishing our mission. Our stated goals reflect the ideas in the mission statement; these ideas guide the development of the goals as we review, meet, and revise them. Each goal is assigned a target date for completion.

Sometimes goals are incomplete because they lack measurable outcomes and timelines. Here are a few examples:

- I will be a caring, competent, and dependable occupational therapy practitioner.

- I will help every client I work with to achieve the highest possible function.
- I will strive for balance in my life, attending to my needs and those of my family.

Use Exercise 3.3 to shift incomplete goals to ones that have achievable and measurable outcomes.

Exercise 3.3. **Revising Goals to Include Measurable, Achievable Behaviors**

In the first column, write the incomplete goals stated earlier in the chapter or write goals of your own that do not define a timeline or lack a way to measure whether you have achieved the goal. Then, restate each goal so that it specifically indicates how to determine when it has been achieved.

Incomplete Goal (Does Not Define How to Measure Achievement or Completion)	Revised Goal (Specifies Identifiable Progress or Completion)

Evaluating Goals Using RUMBA

Good goals require a focus on measurable results and strategic planning. The following five characteristics, abbreviated as RUMBA (Gateley, 2023), will help you evaluate the quality of your goals:

1. **Relevant.** A good goal is based on values that have meaning to you. Your values may drive you to improve professional competency or clinical skills.
2. **Understandable.** A good goal is clearly stated and contains enough details so that you can recognize progress and completion as well as what needs to be done to make the goal happen.
3. **Measurable.** A good goal has specific, expected outcomes and target dates for completion. The outcomes may be in the form of behaviors, performances, or products.
4. **Behavioral.** A good goal focuses on behaviors that can be influenced and changed.
5. **Achievable.** A good goal can be achieved with reasonable effort. It is realistic, motivating, and broken into small action steps that can be completed in the stated completion time.

Use Exercise 3.4 to practice applying RUMBA and identifying good goals.

Exercise 3.4. Identifying Good Goals

For each of the following goals, decide if it meets the RUMBA requirements. In Columns 2 through 6, put a check mark when a goal meets the measurability requirement and a zero (0) when the goal does not. Then revise each of the goals that does not meet all of the RUMBA requirements.

Goal	Relevant	Understandable	Measurable	Behavioral	Achievable
1. Arrive at work every day on time.					
2. Achieve the highest rating on most of my evaluations.					
3. Improve my ability to evaluate clients.					
4. By the end of next week, learn 5 new activities to use when working with stroke clients.					
5. Improve the accuracy of my documentation.					

The following is my revision of each goal so that it meets all of the RUMBA requirements:

1. ____

2. ____

3. ____

4. ____

5. ____

Now, using RUMBA as your guide, create your own personal goals. Use Exercise 3.5 to write your goals. Many fieldwork students benefit from personal goals aimed at nurturing themselves through self-care, stress management, and affirmation to enhance their confidence and self-esteem.

Exercise 3.5. Writing Personal Goals

Write two personal goals that you want to achieve during your fieldwork experience. In Columns 2 through 6, briefly describe how each goal meets each of the RUMBA requirements.

Personal Goal 1	Reasonable	Understand-able	Measurable	Behavioral	Achievable
Personal Goal 2	**Reasonable**	**Understand-able**	**Measurable**	**Behavioral**	**Achievable**

Next, using RUMBA as your guide, create your own professional goals. Many fieldwork students benefit from behavioral goals to enhance their professional interactions, such as handling awkward or uncomfortable conversations and effective communication. Use Exercise 3.6 to write your professional goals.

Exercise 3.6. Writing Professional Goals

Write two professional goals that you want to achieve during fieldwork. In Columns 2 through 6, briefly describe how each goal meets each of the RUMBA requirements.

Professional Goal 1	Reasonable	Understand-able	Measurable	Behavioral	Achievable
Professional Goal 2	**Reasonable**	**Understand-able**	**Measurable**	**Behavioral**	**Achievable**

Talk It Over With Your Fieldwork Supervisor

Consider sharing and discussing your professional goals with your fieldwork supervisor. Let them know what you hope to achieve. This information may help them guide your work and maximize their contributions to your professional growth.

Moving Forward With Your Personal and Professional Goals

> "By the inch, it's a cinch; by the yard, it seems hard; by the mile, it's a trial."
>
> —UNKNOWN

Think of a goal as a destination. Trying to achieve a goal without an action plan to follow is like heading to an unfamiliar location without a map. Some goals are relatively simple and require only a few steps. Others are more complex, require careful planning, and would benefit from help from unfamiliar resources. Long-term goals can be made more manageable and less overwhelming if divided into short-term goals comprising a series of specific smaller steps toward achieving the long-term goal. Such short-term goals provide motivation because one can achieve each step toward the larger goal and experience a sense of progress.

Long- and short-term goals are based on knowing one's personal and professional mission statements. Consider the following professional mission statement from occupational therapy student Felicia: "I will be a caring, competent, dependable occupational therapy practitioner." Fulfilling this mission may necessitate achieving numerous goals that require mastering specialized skills, learning efficient and effective behaviors, and changing long-practiced routines.

Felicia starts her plan off with the following three long-term goals:

1. Improve my oral communication skills.
2. Organize my personal life so I can always be at work on time.
3. Learn to conduct a wider variety of group activities.

Felicia needs to determine how she will know she has achieved these goals by quantifying what success for each one means and determining her timeline for achieving each goal. She can then divide each goal into achievable, measurable steps to complete. Some long-term goals require two or three short-term ones, whereas more complex long-term goals require multiple short-term ones. Short-term goals are usually more specific and less complex than long-term ones, and each short-term goal contributes to achieving the long-term goal. Think of goal setting this way: To easily lift 100 pounds, you have to start with small weights; otherwise, you set yourself up for failure and possibly injury. Using concrete, short-term goals allows you to analyze the whole goal and identify ways to break the long-term goal into short, relevant, understandable, measurable, behavioral, and achievable (i.e., RUMBA) steps.

Leveraging Tools and Resources for Goal Achievement

You can record on a calendar the timeline for achieving goals or use a goal-tracking smartphone app to track your progress. After deciding on a goal, set a completion date on your calendar or in the app. Next, determine the steps toward achieving that goal; these are your short-term goals. Write each to meet the requirements of RUMBA. Then, consider how long each short-term goal will take to achieve, and note on the calendar the completion date of that particular step. Mark a date on the calendar a few days before the completion date with a reminder that you have X numbers of days before completion. Revising completion dates is okay as long as you aren't just delaying doing something. RUMBA helps make the goals concrete—not just another form of New Year's resolutions.

Next, consider what resources may help you achieve your goal. Exhibit 3.1 shows how to evaluate those resources. Returning to the earlier example of Felicia in the previous section, how would this evaluation look with Felicia's goal "Organize my personal life so that I can always be at work on time"? Actions to achieve this goal might include the following:

- Buying a reliable alarm clock or consistently using a smartphone alarm.
- Setting out children's and one's clothing the night before they are needed.
- Packing lunches, or breakfast to-go, the night before needed.
- Requesting help from family members to make lunches.
- Going to bed by 10:30 p.m. Setting a phone alarm or smartwatch notification as a reminder.
- Saving your favorite TV shows to view or stream on the weekend. You can binge-watch later as a reward for adhering to your action steps.

Next, referring again to the example of Felicia, use Exercise 3.7 to develop a plan of action for her goal "Organize my personal life so that I can always be at work on time." Then complete Exercise 3.8 to create your own professional action plan.

EXHIBIT 3.1. Finding Resources to Achieve Goals

Important Questions to Ask	Possible Resources
What information do I need? Examples of information needed could include: • Directions or tutorial videos for beginning an assessment, using an evaluation, or conducting an activity • Instructions for using a piece of equipment	Find resources by asking the next two questions.
Where can I look? Who can I ask for ideas?	• Internet • Library • Textbooks • Class notes • Other professionals and staff with whom I will work

Who can help me? Who could be sources of information?	• Other professionals • Classmates • Friends • Family members and relatives

Exercise 3.7. Creating an Action Plan for Felicia's Arrival to the Fieldwork Site

List 5 more steps or actions that support Felicia's arrival on time to her fieldwork site every day:

1. ______________________________

2. ______________________________

3. ______________________________

4. ______________________________

5. ______________________________

Now, using Exercise 3.8, create a professional action plan for your short- and long-terms goals.

Exercise 3.8. Creating a Professional Action Plan

Create a plan for one of your professional goals. Then break that goal down into a series of short-term goals.

Long-term goal: ______________________________

Targeted completion date: ______________________________

Short-term goal 1: ______________________________

Completion date: ______________________________

Short-term goal 2: ______________________________

Completion date: ______________________________

Short-term goal 3: ______________________________

Completion date: ______________________________

Short-term goal 4: ______________________________

Completion date: ______________________________

Talk it Over With Your Fieldwork Supervisor

Consider sharing your action plans with your fieldwork supervisor. Do they have suggestions or ideas they personally use? Offer some ideas that you've considered to make your action plan more successful, and learn to accept suggestions. You may not use the suggestions, but those ideas may lead you to others that work for you.

Exploring Habits That Help, Habits That Hinder

Poor habits can hold us back from performing at our highest level (Graybiel & Smith, 2014). Fieldwork is an excellent time to review your habits and identify any that might prevent you from realizing your full potential as an occupational therapy practitioner. For example, personal habits like procrastinating or overloading yourself with too many responsibilities can interfere with your desire to help others. Good habits, on the other hand, can be powerful forces for developing professional competence. They contribute to your efficiency and make it easier to do what is necessary to achieve the goals you have selected (Graybiel & Smith, 2014).

If something you've done is not your fault, how can you be responsible for improving yourself? Through honest self-appraisal and acceptance of responsibility, you empower yourself to change. You identify the problem, work to make the necessary changes, and then give yourself credit for a worthy accomplishment.

Some poor habits have served useful purposes in the past. Changing them, though, may require you to find other ways to meet your needs or substitute positive behaviors. For example, a person wants to lose weight but overeats to alleviate anxiety. The anxiety is unlikely to disappear on its own. Finding alternative ways to lessen anxiety may be necessary before weight loss can be successful. Understanding the motivation for habits not in one's best interest can promote and support behavioral changes. Try not to get hung up on blame or how the habit became part of your response to things. Instead, focus on the future, the changes you can control, and promotion of your success. That is self-empowerment! Use Exercise 3.9 to examine one of your bad habits, then create a goal to empower yourself and change your professional performance.

Habits can be difficult to change. Be willing to be both persistent and patient—patient with yourself just as you would be reasonable with clients and patient as they make small steps toward learning new routines. New habits are not established and old ones are not broken overnight. Backsliding happens, but that is not a reason to give up. It took time to learn a bad habit, and it will take time to change it. Plan rewards to congratulate yourself for achieving the small steps toward the larger goal.

Exercise 3.9. **Changing a Bad Habit**

Create a goal to help you change a bad habit, or create a new habit—a good one—that can help make your fieldwork experience more successful.

1. Describe a habit (bad or good):

____

____

2. Write a goal for this habit:

____

____

3. If you are changing a habit, does this habit fit a personal need? Can you meet this need in more productive ways? If so, what are they?

____

____

4. Set a target completion date. Make your timeline reasonable to maximize your potential for success.

____

____

5. Break your goal into small action steps—as many as needed so each is not too complex to concretely measure and to be achievable.

____

____

Staying Motivated

Student life has built-in requirements and deadlines. Assignments have due dates, and examinations are given at specific times. During fieldwork, you have more freedom and personal responsibility. If your skills need improving, there are no instructors, laboratory sessions, or quizzes to motivate you to work on them. Motivating yourself and finding the resources you need to learn is up to you. The fieldwork supervisor may act as your coach, but following through is also up to you. Internal motivation can be strengthened by being clear about what is important and staying focused on your goals. Accomplishing your plan is an empowering and joyful experience for both you and your clients. When you turned in assignments in class, you received feedback through grades and comments. In the clinic, you may frequently have to provide your own feedback as well as give feedback to your clients. Less feedback from others does not mean no feedback. In the clinic, you are more likely to hear negative feedback when something doesn't go as expected than congratulations when things are successful. Success is the expected outcome. Clients never ask to see your transcripts. They look at what they can achieve because of your interventions and often have trouble seeing success unless you can set measurable goals to show them their success. If you have done your best, notice yourself. Give yourself credit! Motivation that comes from within, combined with meeting your own expectations, can bring greater satisfaction to your work and personal life. Set measurable goals and congratulate yourself on your achievements. When others notice, it's a bonus.

Creating Client Goals

Creating goals for clients is an essential part of the therapeutic process. Long- and short-term goals provide the basis for therapeutic plans and the monitoring of client progress: for you, for third-party payers, and for motivating clients.

The ability to distinguish between your goals for the client and the client's stated goals is an important professional skill. Client goals are stated in terms of the expected behavioral outcomes of the client, not the occupational therapy practitioner. Using the RUMBA characteristics to evaluate the goals helps illustrate the difference. Is the goal measurable regarding the client's change in observable performance? Can the behavior be described as something the client can do as an observable change? New practitioners sometimes confuse client goals with the practitioner's actions or behaviors related to the client. Take another look at what occupational therapist Elena says in the quote near the beginning of this chapter. Her goal, "Complete patient evaluation," is what she will do, not what the client will do. Table 3.1 offers additional examples of the client's goals compared with the practitioner's goals for the client.

TABLE 3.1. Client Goals Compared With the Occupational Therapy Practitioner's Goals

Client Goals	Practitioner's Goals Related to the Client
Put on and take off shoes and socks by the end of 4 treatment sessions.	Select appropriate assistive devices based on client's skills and teach client how to use the devices.
Prepare a meal independently from a wheelchair to feed their family of four within 1 month.	Work with client to increase upper extremity range of motion and strength to enable meal preparation from a wheelchair.
Cooperate with other group members by not interrupting when others are speaking.	Work with client to control impulsive behaviors.

When writing client goals, ask the following questions to see if the goals meet the RUMBA characteristics:

- Relevant
  - Are they based on what is important to the client?
  - Do they meet the client's needs?
  - Will they help the client achieve the highest level of function possible?
  - Are they appropriate for the client's diagnosis
  - Will they meet the requirements of the third-party payer?

- Understandable
  - Are the goals clear to both the client and the occupational therapy practitioner?
  - Do the client's family members understand the goals?
  - Are the goals clear and written such that they are acceptable to the third-party payer?
- Measurable
  - What must the client do to demonstrate achievement of the goal?
  - How will achievement be measured quantitatively?
  - What are the target dates for completion?
  - Does the client know exactly what they must do to achieve the goal?
- Behavioral
  - What behavior will the client demonstrate?
  - What changes in behavior will occur?
- Achievable
  - Given the referral or diagnosis, can the client be expected to achieve the goal?
  - Are the goals too difficult or too easy?
  - Is there sufficient time? Equipment? Are other necessary resources available?

Just as values form the foundation of your own goals, you must consider and respect the client's values when creating their goals. The occupational therapy practitioner is responsible for listening to the client and asking questions to learn what is important to that client. They can then plan meaningful tasks to motivate the client to take an active role in the therapeutic process. The practitioner must be hopeful but realistic about what can be expected to be accomplished.

Long-term goals for clients may involve achievement of occupational performance or participation, whereas short-term goals consist of specific functional skills needed to accomplish the long-term goal. The goal of independently preparing a meal is long term, requiring several specific skills (short-term goals), such as the ability to

- open and reach into the refrigerator and cupboards;
- use assistive devices to grasp and place materials on the kitchen counter when necessary;
- grasp and manipulate cooking and eating utensils;
- address safety issues related to turning the stove on and off; and
- move hot pans safely between stove, counters, and table.

Creating appropriate client goals often requires input from others, such as the client's family members, your clinical supervisor, and the clients themselves. Good communication and collaboration skills are necessary to plan client goals effectively. Fieldwork offers many opportunities to practice these essential skills.

Talk It Over With Your Fieldwork Supervisor

Talk with your supervisor about how they plan client goals. You may wish to ask these questions:

- How do they encourage client involvement in creating goals?
- What advice can you [fieldwork supervisor] give you about engaging clients in goal setting and using RUMBA criteria for measurable goals?

Summary

The exercises in this chapter are designed to help you identify and focus on goals that are important to you and to the client. Developing specific and well-planned personal, professional, and client goals can maximize your fieldwork experiences and foster future career success. Written goals can help your clinical fieldwork supervisors better support your development as a clinician and help you realize your potential.

Differentiating *your* goals from your *clients'* goals is a mark of professional competence. Fieldwork will offer you many opportunities to sharpen these skills.

References

Agency for Healthcare Research and Quality. (2024). *Consider culture: Tool 10.* https://www.ahrq.gov/health-literacy/improve/precautions/tool10.html

Almutairi, R. L., Aditya, R. S., Kodriyah, L., Yusuf, A., Solikhah, F. K., Al Razeeni, D. M., & Kotijah, S. (2022). Analysis of organizational culture factors that influence the performance of health care professionals: A literature review. *Journal of Public Health in Africa, 13*(Suppl. 2), 2415. https://doi.org/10.4081/jphia.2022.2415

American Psychological Association. (2018). *Group pressure.* https://dictionary.apa.org/group-pressure

Ethics Resource Center. (2014). *Peer influence: How others impact the way we behave.* https://www.ethics.org/wp-content/uploads/2014-ECI-WP-Peer-Influence-How-Others-Impact-the-Way-We-Behave.pdf

Gateley, C. (2023). *Documentation manual for occupational therapy* (5th ed.). Rutledge Press.

Graybiel, A. M., & Smith, K. S. (2014). Good habits, bad habits. *Scientific American, 310*(6), 38–43. https://doi.org/10.1038/scientificamerican0614-38

Gurung, R. A. R. (2019). Cultural influences on health. In K. D. Keith (Ed.), *Cross-cultural psychology.* https://doi.org/9781119519348/10.1002.ch21

Mannion, R., & Davies, H. (2018). Understanding organisational culture for healthcare quality improvement. *British Medical Journal, 363,* k4907. https://doi.org/10.1136/bmj.k4907

Social Value International. (n.d.). *What is social value?* https://www.socialvalueint.org/what-is-social-value

Chapter 4

Time Management and Self-Care Strategies

TOPICS

- Managing the gift of time
- Matching your goals to dates in your calendar
- Being there!
- Planning ahead to lessen stress
- Making lists work for you
- Addressing the procrastination problem
- Maximizing your focus: Determining your most productive times
- Becoming an efficient practitioner
- Developing effective work habits
- Combatting time thieves
- Learning to say "no"
- Making the most of leisure time
- Applying strategies for personal organization

I started getting better when I began to keep a calendar and a schedule. It was those daily journals that I thought were so stupid in my rehab treatment. You see, it's normal to have a calendar and write stuff down. No one can keep it all in their own head, especially me, because I injured my brain. But I actually do more and do it more efficiently now because I've learned to keep a calendar and make daily lists.

—DAN, survivor of a brain injury

Managing the Gift of Time

The way we spend our time determines the quality of our lives. Effectively using and enjoying the hours allotted to us influences our personal and professional success. Modern life places huge demands on our time. Occupational therapy practitioners are busy, whether attending school, raising a family, completing fieldwork, or working on the job. In a health care environment that relies on health insurance reimbursement, time has significant financial implications (Bennett et al., 2019). One study on clinician perceptions in inpatient rehabilitation found that rising productivity standards are affecting health care professionals' perceived ability to provide quality care, and the accompanying time pressure is increasing unprofessional behaviors (Bennett et al., 2019). Productivity standards and reimbursement realities can present challenges for fieldwork educators balancing productivity demands while supervising and supporting a student through their daily grind (Ozelle et al., 2015).

Some students may also feel overwhelmed by the demands of fieldwork, particularly in Level II fieldwork. They typically have had to change locations, adjust their routines, and rearrange personal priorities to accommodate the new schedule of fieldwork work days, locations, and travel time and to achieve success in several new clinical sites. Remember: The goal of fieldwork is to introduce you to the variety of occupational therapy practice settings, allowing you to become a safe and efficient entry-level practitioner. Fieldwork is the bridge between academic work and professional practice that makes a difference in people's lives. This chapter focuses on ways to help you manage your time so you can both enjoy and profit from the learning opportunities presented in fieldwork.

Matching Your Goals to Dates in Your Calendar

Time is the most precious resource for good planning. It may seem easy to wait until the last minute to do something, but the less stressful plan means organizing—like gathering the necessary documents needed for fieldwork—well ahead of time. Making a list of things you must do before starting fieldwork is like planning for a trip. What do you need for a successful "trip" to your fieldwork site? As mentioned in Chapter 3, consider a goal to be a destination. The intention of using a long-term goal is not to put off what needs to be done; rather, a long-term goal identifies more complex things that need to be accomplished so that you can break that goal into smaller, more manageable steps (i.e., short-term goals).

Recording goals and their completion dates in a planner (see Part V of this book) or on your smartphone app can help you better use your time. The planner or smartphone apps are useful tools to help you organize your daily life as well as help you increase your personal and professional efficiency and productivity. By jotting down your goals, action steps, and target completion dates, you can make your planner serve as your road map to success in fieldwork, step-by-step. Some complex goals have many parts, so breaking a long-term goal into smaller ones makes the road to success seem less complicated because doing so provides visible steps toward the ultimate goal. Think of it this way: Like the most massive computers that are programmed in bits, "bites" (i.e. bytes), and nibbles, we set a goal and achieve it by breaking it down into smaller, achievable steps—our personal bits, bites, and nibbles. Subdividing goals can help you in these ways:

- Large goals and projects seem less overwhelming when broken down into smaller components.
- You need only take small amounts of time to make progress toward achieving the small steps. Focus on the inch, not the mile.
- You can keep a journal of written and documented achievement to encourage further action. Revisiting your journal can remind you that you have progressed and provide personal satisfaction and motivation toward continued achievement.

Review the professional action plan you created in Chapter 3 (see Exercise 3.8). Did you assign completion dates for each short-term goal and write them in a calendar on those dates? If you didn't, make your goals and timelines a reality by adding them to the calendar pages in the planner part of this book. Goals without timelines are like daydreams: "want-to-haves" that may be unrealistic. Exercise 4.1 will help you plan your way to success by creating small but achievable goals.

Exercise 4.1. Plan Your Way to Success by Creating Achievable Steps

For this exercise, use the short-term goals you wrote in Chapter 3 (see Exercise 3.8) on creating a professional action plan to break your goals into achievable steps. Usually, a goal takes 2 to 4 actions steps, but possibly more depending on the complexity of the goal. Transfer the action steps and completion dates onto the calendar pages in your planner. You can have more than four action steps.

Long-term goal: ______ Completion date: ______		
Short-Term Goal and Completion Date	**Action Steps**	**Target Completion Date**
Short-term goal 1:	1. ______ 2. ______ 3. ______ 4. ______	
Short-term goal 2:	1. ______ 2. ______ 3. ______ 4. ______	

Short-term goal 3:	1. ______ 2. ______ 3. ______ 4. ______	
Short-term goal 4:	1. ______ 2. ______ 3. ______ 4. ______	

Now think about what you need to do to achieve each short-term goal. How can the goals be further broken down into bite-sized portions? Returning to the example of Felicia, an occupational therapy student introduced in Chapter 3 who was working on her goals, consider the following actions that Felicia could complete in short periods to work on her goal "Learn to conduct a wider variety of group activities":

- Review textbooks and notes from classes.
- Read a short informational article or book chapter about group activities.
- Observe an experienced practitioner conducting a group session.
- Email an instructor from school to discuss or request information about group activities.
- Do an internet search for ideas or start a shared folder with classmates to exchange group activity ideas.
- Draft group protocols with activities that include the activity's purpose and required materials.
- Join an interest group on social media or through the American Occupational Therapy Association where you can exchange ideas with peers and experienced practitioners.

Being There!

During fieldwork and on the job, knowing exactly when and where you should be is extremely important. Clients depend on you to provide services in a timely manner. Colleagues depend on you to carry your share of the workload. Being *on-site, on time, every day,* and *professionally documenting client interventions* are top priorities of the successful occupational therapy practitioner.

Your work schedule is one of the first things to check when you begin working at each fieldwork setting. Use the calendar section in Part V of this book or a smartphone app to record the essentials, including, but not limited to, the following:

- your weekly and daily schedule and your arrival and departure times
- the name and phone number of the person to contact if you will be late or absent; remember that being late or absent can disrupt others' schedules
- the dates of meetings and any other known activities you are expected to attend
- a regular time for meeting with your fieldwork supervisor to talk about your progress and any problems that have occurred, and to learn from your supervisor's experience by discussing topics you list in planning for this meeting.

Adult student learners typically have many responsibilities in addition to those related to their education. A key to successfully balancing multiple priorities is *planning.* Anticipate in advance what might cause you to be late or unable to attend your fieldwork assignment (see Exercise 4.2 for more information on overcoming obstacles.) The following actions can help relieve stress and ensure regular attendance:

- Make arrangements for reliable child care, including pickup plans for emergencies, such as illness of the caregiver or the child.
- Secure dependable transportation and learn about alternative means, such as public transportation, ride shares, or carpooling with colleagues at the fieldwork site.
- Arrange for stable housing. If you are staying in temporary accommodations, have backup plans if it becomes necessary to move.
- Set up alternative care arrangements for anyone who depends on you for assistance, such as an older family member, children, or a family member with a disability.
- Take care of routine medical and dental checkups ahead of time to minimize routine health care during fieldwork and to prevent personal health emergencies. Emergencies occur even with the best planning, so have a plan to respond.

Exercise 4.2. **Overcoming Obstacles: A Personal Plan**

Use the following chart to identify and plan preventive measures for your own potential obstacles. In the "Useful Resources" column, note names, phone numbers, websites, email addresses, and more for easy access.

Personal Obstacles	Prevention Plans	Useful Resources

Planning Ahead to Lessen Stress

Here are other ideas to help you stay organized, plan your time efficiently, and control your daily life. Becoming efficient at handling routine tasks can enable you to devote more time to major priorities and unplanned events in daily life. Start by marking the dates of events you don't want to forget, such as:

- academic paperwork deadlines and method for submission
- National Board for Certification in Occupational Therapy examination application deadline and paperwork needed to complete the application
- renewal dates for fieldwork compliance requirements, such as CPR certification or tuberculosis skin tests
- graduation-related deadlines and events
- birthdays
- anniversaries
- appointments
- payment due dates
- social events.

Record events in your planner or smartphone app to track important activities that include your family members and friends, such as children's athletic events and school activities, a spouse's company dinner, or events for which you might need to bring something. Use highlighters or color code to draw attention to important dates or critical deadlines. "Alert" and other electronic notifications on calendar events can help. You can usually put two such alerts on a single event—what I (Bonnie, the author of this book) call first: "Get dressed or change clothes" and second: "Get out to the car now!" In addition to everyday use, develop the habit of reviewing your digital or planner calendar at the beginning of each month, each week, and each morning to monitor your progress toward goals.

Making Lists Work for You

Time management specialists have suggested that writing prioritized daily to-do lists is the single best technique for maximizing one's use of time (Schrager, 2022). Along with errands and appointments, include in your to-do lists actions that will contribute to achieving your goals. Doing so can help prevent the goals that are considered short-term urgent from getting in the way of steps to complete the long-term important ones.

At the beginning or end of each day, write your list on your calendar in the "Tasks for Today" section (see the calendar pages in Part V) and then prioritize the list in order of importance. The focus of each day's efforts should be on completing the most important items first, providing concrete inspiration, and freeing up your energy toward completing the remaining goals. If the unexpected happens—which it often does—you have at least taken care of the prioritized items by planning. At the end of each day, check off the items completed and move the remaining, incomplete ones to the next day. Reward yourself by seeing what you've accomplished; it doesn't always seem like much has happened until you review your list!

For the next 2 weeks, write a daily to-do list. Effective list makers often add items they know will be done to add to the feeling of successful completion or concretely look at all they have been doing. Making lists is about more than just things you might forget to do! It gives you concrete, visible accomplishments. At the end of a 2-week period, evaluate how writing a daily to-do list helped with the following:

- prioritization and accomplishment of tasks
- effective use of time
- completion of action steps
- achievement of goals.

Talk It Over With Your Fieldwork Supervisor

Talk with your supervisor at each site about prioritizing your tasks. Discuss strategies they have developed that help them determine what is most important and ask how they decide the order in which tasks should be completed.

Addressing the Procrastination Problem

Putting off what needs to be done is a common habit and can cause unnecessary stress. Research shows that procrastination arises from multiple personal and situational factors, including one's personality traits, task characteristics (e.g., ambiguous instructions, lack of incentives), and environmental traits (e.g., tempting social media, fun distractors; Hen & Goroshit, 2018). If procrastination is a problem for you, try to identify your reasons for putting things off. You can then begin dealing with the root of the problem root and form new habits. Look at Exhibit 4.1: Do any of the reasons for procrastinating apply to you? Can you identify a pattern of behavior?

EXHIBIT 4.1. Procrastination: Reasons and Remedies

Reasons for Procrastinating	Suggested Remedies
Some tasks just seem overwhelming. I don't know where to start.	• Gather needed information. • Begin with a small, easy task to complete. • Break the project into smaller, more manageable portions. • Write a plan of action. • Ask for guidance from a supervisor, colleague, or friend who is qualified to help.

I'm unfamiliar with the task. I'm not sure what to do. I'm not really interested in doing it.	• Build in rewards for work completed. • Visualize both starting and completing tasks. • Think in terms of benefits to be gained once the task is completed.
I'm afraid I'll make a mistake or fail completely.	• Consider that failure to act at all may mean loss of a learning opportunity. • Try positive self-talk to boost your confidence. • Ask for help or seek more information, directions, or clarification. • Assess your readiness for the task. Do you need more information?
I just have too much to do.	• "No" is a complete sentence. Learn to say "no" to requests you really don't have time to do. Saying "yes" and not following through is worse than saying "no" in the first place. • Check to see if you're using the time you have as efficiently as you can. • Review your priorities.
I can't really work until the last minute when there's pressure to meet a deadline.	• Set your own deadlines to create a sense of "controlled urgency." • Consider the benefits of working at a steady pace: fewer frantic moments, time to deal with the unexpected, higher quality product or outcome.

Sometimes, procrastination comes from fear of failure and difficulty managing one's anxiety (Hen & Goroshit, 2018). By avoiding a task, you temporarily avoid feedback and the learning experience that comes with it. By recognizing fear and acknowledging your anxiety, you can develop strategies to handle your fear in positive ways. Good self-care and anxiety management starts with you. The fieldwork environment is new and novel. It can feel scarier than the classroom, lab, or simulation center. Most students feel more anxious on fieldwork rotations than they do in the classroom (Cornine, 2020; Moscaritolo, 2009). It's best to build your anxiety management toolbox and skills to use that toolbox well before you start Level II fieldwork. Don't wait until you enter the building on day one to try out anxiety management techniques like deep breathing, mindfulness, meditation, and positive self-affirmations (Cornine, 2020). It's too hard to start using those techniques your first week. Rather, practice anxiety management strategies throughout your academic program, so it feels natural and accessible when you're having a hard day and find yourself avoiding the task or feedback at hand. Once you retrain your mind, then you can master your time and the tasks before you. Research shows that good time and task management enhances people's job performance, academic achievement, and well-being (Aeon et al., 2021). Breaking tasks into achievable steps linked with a timeline is the age-old solution to organizing and managing one's time (Brill, 2023). Just as occupational therapy practitioners learn to set long-term and short-term goals for clients, we need to apply these same techniques to our own lives: Set goals realistically, organize what we need to achieve the steps toward these goals, delegate where possible, and trade guilt for action toward goals. Writing lists helps make the actions, steps, and sequences concrete. Electronic devices and apps can be set to remind us of timing and action steps.

Without time management, we cannot apply other intervention skills in time and sequence. Written organization helps us avoid strategies that can take too long or that appear disorganized; writing down goals and steps helps us clarify specific sequencing and avoid missing or incomplete steps. Facing fears head-on, checking to see if the fear really makes sense, and brainstorming ways to manage anxiety can be wonderfully self-energizing. Overcoming obstacles (see Exercise 4.2) that limit the effective use of time is a key factor in achieving professional and personal success.

Maximizing Your Focus: Determining Your Most Productive Times

You may be a "morning person"—someone who steps out of bed at 5 a.m. ready to start the day. Or maybe you're a "night owl" who becomes most productive after many of us have headed for bed. Each of us has a biological rhythm that determines our most productive times. You can improve your efficiency by identifying and taking advantage of these times.

Of course, work schedules do not always correspond with our bodies' preferences! However, being aware of your "best times" regarding mental concentration and physical energy can help you plan effectively and make decisions when you have a choice. You can also share this insight with your fieldwork educator who might be able to adapt to your temporal rhythms. For example, if you feel sharper at the beginning of the day, then maybe that's the best time for debriefing the previous work day with your supervisor or completing cognitively demanding tasks. If you can't concentrate during the evening hours, then set aside time on the weekend to study and review information for your fieldwork placement. Track your energy levels during a few typical days. Can you identify ways to take advantage of your rhythms?

Becoming an Efficient Practitioner

Today's occupational therapy practitioners must strive for balance when working with clients who want—and deserve—caring attention. At the same time, practitioners have demanding schedules that require high efficiency and productivity. The ability to focus on the task and move along without seeming to rush is a valuable skill. The new practitioner can use several techniques to maximize the time spent with each client:

- Be prepared before meeting with clients. Gather necessary equipment and supplies ahead of time. Review charts and diagnoses.
- Let clients know how much time you have available. This way, you won't have to leave just as they are about to ask you questions or share important information.

- Explain the purpose of occupational therapy and the benefits to clients.
- Ask the client if they have any special needs so you can address those needs first.
- Briefly outline the action plan so the client will know what to expect.
- Focus fully on the client and listen carefully. Active listening also improves the quality of time spent with clients and others.
- Use questions and feedback to prevent misunderstandings resulting in wasted time. Be specific and clear in your questions. You don't often have time for open-ended questions, especially with clients who may respond tangentially with unnecessary distractions. You need to be specific to get the needed information quickly.
- Demonstrate a pleasant demeanor that conveys interest in the other person.
- Face the other person and make eye contact when you are speaking. Avoid postures that make you appear in a hurry to leave.
- Work as calmly as possible. Doing so puts others at ease, helps you avoid mistakes, and doesn't escalate the anxiety that clients often feel.
- Stay mindful and present in the moment and pay attention to the task. Avoid being distracted by past or future events. The client deserves your full attention.
- Let the client know what to expect in the next session so that they can be prepared.

You can also apply many of these techniques to your communication with colleagues and supervisors.

Developing Effective Work Habits

In addition to maximizing the quality of client contact time, you can manage the time designated to other work tasks to help relieve some of the time crunch and feeling of "Where DID the afternoon go?" One of the first things to do when you arrive at each fieldwork site is to get to know the location and the procedures. If complete information is not provided to you, don't hesitate to ask. Knowing a facility's ins and outs will save time later.

Use the at-a-glance checklist in Exhibit 4.2 to help organize information and locate needed materials while completing your fieldwork.

EXHIBIT 4.2. Compilation of Necessary Fieldwork Information: At-a-Glance Checklist

Item	Location of Item	Comments
Supplies (consumables)		
Equipment and storage		
Forms		

Policy and procedure manuals		
Instructions for equipment		
Library and location of resource materials		
Other necessary items or information		

In addition to this checklist, try the following helpful time management and organizational strategies for busy professionals:

- **Write a to-do list.** This is a powerful time management tool if used consistently.
- **Cluster your tasks.** Schedule tasks together when they use the same equipment and materials. In one sitting, make phone calls or complete online tasks of paying bills and updating your calendar while at the computer. Plan errands so that you can reduce the number of trips.
- **Do it once.** Deal with paperwork or email as you receive it. When appropriate, write memos or add sticky notes to the paperwork. Strive to complete tasks correctly the first time so you won't have to repeat them.
- **Document immediately.** Delaying documentation increases the risk of errors or omissions. Doing so can also take more time as you try to recall details. Remember that client charts are legal documents that courts or lawyers can later subpoena.
- **Use downtime.** Use waiting time to read, think, problem solve, or write a list. These moments can add up in a day! Keep work handy by saving information that you need to review on your smartphone or tablet (except for information protected by the Health Insurance Portability and Accountability Act of 1996 [P. L. 104-191]). Use time waiting for a doctor's appointment to look up treatment ideas or review the scientific literature.
- **Put it back where it belongs.** Help yourself and those with whom you work to be efficient. Don't waste time looking for where you left something or explaining to coworkers where you left items that they need *now*. Return materials and equipment to their storage places. Keep your workspace clean and organized.
- **Deal efficiently with interruptions.** Interruptions—common in the workplace—can derail the best-laid plans. Learn to handle interruptions tactfully and refocus on your task. Say a coworker wants to share personal news with you. You might respond in a friendly way to convey that you are too busy to talk at that time: "That really sounds interesting, but I have to get this report finished. I'd like to hear about it at lunch after I finish this documentation."
- **Take notes.** Keep a clipboard, notebooks, or a digital notepad on your smartphone or tablet handy so you can take notes throughout the day. Check with your

supervisor to ensure it's okay to use an electronic device like tablet or smartphone to take notes; it could be interpreted as "off-task" behavior, depending on the context. Writing down questions you want ask your supervisor, a main point covered in an important conversation, or a phone message helps prevent backtracking, asking the same question again, or just plain forgetting information.

- **Observe others.** Identify professionals in your fieldwork settings who are good time managers and observe their work habits. Are they using techniques you can apply?

Complete Exercise 4.3 to discover other strategies that can help you work more efficiently.

Exercise 4.3. **Techniques for Increasing Your Efficiency at Work**

Based on your particular fieldwork assignments, develop a list of techniques for yourself that might increase your work efficiency.

1. ______________________________

2. ______________________________

3. ______________________________

4. ______________________________

5. ______________________________

Combatting Time Thieves

Daily life is full of interruptions, habits, and distractions that steal time. Observe your habits and how you spend time during school or work. Consider keeping a time diary for a few days. In this diary, account for each 30-minute interval. Take a few moments at the end of each day to review the diary and identify things that waste your time (see Exercise 4.4). The following are common workplace examples of problems and possible solutions. See if any of these problems apply to you:

- Spending too much time socializing with coworkers
  Solution: Plan a time to get together at the end of the day or off-site in a relaxing setting.
- Feeling overwhelmed by documentation
  Solution: Create a note-writing template or checklist to help you gather information more efficiently and effectively and also to ensure you're completing the necessary steps for filing paperwork and billing.

- Spending too much time on your phone
  Solution: Use a timer to monitor the length of your calls, FaceTime, or social media usage.

Exercise 4.4. **Time Thieves**

Record your own time thieves and possible solutions. Note any resources that may be helpful.

Problem	Possible Solutions	Helpful Resources

Talk It Over With Your Fieldwork Supervisor

Ask your supervisor at each site to share time-saving tips and techniques they learned from their own experience. Also ask:

- What advice can they offer about working efficiently and in a caring manner?
- How do they schedule their work to ensure the essential tasks are completed?

Learning to Say "No"

Learning to say "no" to requests in your personal and social life that put additional but unnecessary stress on your time and energy during fieldwork can help reduce feelings of overload. Life is full of demands, and an inability to realistically assess one's capabilities and limitations is a common cause of stress (Dierdorff, 2020). Establishing boundaries is part of personal and professional growth. When you honor the fact that time is a limited resource, then you can truly learn how to wisely arrange your time (Dierdorff, 2020).

When making choices about how much you decide to take on, ask yourself the following questions:

- Your fieldwork performance is a major priority and is essential to your professional development. Success in fieldwork is critical to passing the certification examination and getting a job. You are nearing completion of your education and professional training. Will the task or activity you are considering help or hinder your reaching that goal?
- Will the task or activity contribute to achieving your professional goal?
- What are the likely consequences of turning down the request or invitation?
- If related to a job not associated with occupational therapy, can you take on one more student loan or request emergency funds to free up time, actions that can contribute to your experience and success in fieldwork?

  It can be difficult to take on more student loan debt, but after graduating, your income will increase dramatically, including your ability to pay off student loans! You only get the fieldwork experience once. Make the most of this culminating educational experience. And, yes, this was my (Bonnie, co-author of this book) quandary and agony, and the ability to focus on my fieldwork experience contributed to my success as an occupational therapist and to the writing of this book. Make the most of your fieldwork!

When it is hard to say "no," remember that it is more considerate to say "no" to a request at the beginning than to promise to do something and then be unable to follow through. Not fulfilling promises can produce more stress than turning down requests.

Striving for Work–Life Balance

Although you may not have as much free time as you'd like, it's important to find a balance between fieldwork and self-care. Free time during fieldwork is likely precious and scarce, so you'll want to purposely plan activities that are relaxing and help you fill your proverbial cup. Research shows that taking time for leisure as a full-time student improves one's quality of life, reduces stress, and increases overall satisfaction with the learning experience (Terzi et al., 2024). Choose activities that contribute to your physical and mental well-being.

Ask yourself: What are my leisure choices? How do I relax? An activity that can feel like work to one person and might be relaxing for someone else. Using free time for self-care and leisure can enhance your focus, boost your immune system, and increase energy for fieldwork. Use your digital or paper planner to schedule time for yourself. Even a walk or meditation during the work day counts toward your "you" time.

If incorporating leisure is not enough and you are feeling very overwhelmed, then it's time to check in with your stress levels and reach out for support. No one expects you to do hard things alone, and fieldwork can be hard. You have an entire village behind you that consists of your academic advisor and fieldwork coordinator, your peers and classmates, and your support network. It's okay to ask for help and talk things out with your trusted support system. As an academic fieldwork coordinator, I (Jami, co-author of this book) never want students to suffer in silence. Fieldwork can be a tough experience, so let your support system do what they do best and support you. Also, your trusted academic team may have additional resources, such as access to counselors or career coaches.

You must process a lot of feelings and experiences during fieldwork. Try incorporating journaling, meditation, and self-reflection as regular practices. It's also perfectly acceptable to work with a professional counselor or therapist to process emotions and experiences. Mental health professionals can support hardworking yet stressed-out fieldwork students to manage stress, build executive functioning strategies (e.g., how to go about the work day more effectively), and cope with big feelings (e.g., grief after losing a client, distress with a fast-paced learning environment). Your self-care is critical to your success as a future occupational therapy practitioner. We become occupational therapists and occupational therapy assistants to help others, but we're not always the best at helping ourselves. Prioritize self-care so you can thrive as a future provider.

Applying Strategies for Personal Organization

Staying organized during a busy time in life when you are finishing academic work and fieldwork is challenging. Effective organizational techniques can help you save time and energy and put you in control rather than having external circumstances drain your energy. In the blank spaces in Exercise 4.5, jot down ideas specific to your fieldwork experiences on how the stated technique might work for you.

Exercise 4.5. **Organizational Techniques to Save Time and Energy**

Technique	How Would This Technique Work for You?
Keep resources handy: Carry your planner or binder in which you gather and organize information and resources.	
Take notes: Write down useful information and reminders in your planner/binder.	
Be prepared: Carry supplies you may need during the day in a tote bag, tool belt, or rolling bag and restock it as needed.	
Keep things in designated places: Avoid wasting time and energy looking for things.	
Encourage promptness: Set timers on your watch as reminders.	

Add your own strategies:	
Organizational strategy	**How to implement this strategy**

Summary

Making the best use of your time can have a major effect on your fieldwork success. Developing personal organizational strategies and using a calendar with reminders can maximize your learning and increase your productivity. You are also likely to experience less stress because these tools help you to plan and stay on top of a busy schedule. Less stress can increase the benefits and enjoyment you receive from the fieldwork experience.

Fieldwork is more than an opportunity to expand your learning and receive supervision of how you apply what you have been learning in academic courses. Fieldwork is your opportunity to observe and work with occupational therapy practitioners who can provide references related to your therapeutic skills—how you treat clients professionally and as people in crisis. Drop your personal crises at the door. Plan ahead to keep them from distracting you and preventing you from making creative plans and interventions for your clients. Focus on your clients' occupational needs by planning for your own success—and de-stress.

References

Aeon, B., Faber, A., & Panaccio, A. (2021). Does time management work? A meta-analysis. *PLOS One, 16*(1), e0245066. https://doi.org/10.1371/journal.pone.0245066

Bennett, L. E., Jewell, V. D., Scheirton, L., McCarthy, M., & Muir, B. C. (2019). Productivity standards and the impact on quality of care: A national survey of inpatient rehabilitation professionals. *Open Journal of Occupational Therapy, 7*(4), 1–11. https://doi.org/10.15453/2168-6408.1598

Brill, O. (2023). *Mastering time management skills: The essential guide.* https://www.adcore.com/blog/mastering-time-management-skills-the-essential-guide/

Cornine, A. (2020). Reducing nursing student anxiety in the clinical setting: An integrative review. *Nursing Education Perspectives, 41*(4), 229–234. https://doi.org/10.1097/01.NEP.0000000000000633

Dierdorff, E. C. (2020). *Time management is about more than life hacks.* Harvard Business Review. https://hbr.org/2020/01/time-management-is-about-more-than-life-hacks

Health Insurance Portability and Accountability Act of 1996 (HIPAA), Pub. L. 104–191, 42 U.S.C. § 300gg, 29 U.S.C §§ 1181–1183, and 42 U.S.C. §§ 1320d–1320d9.

Hen, M., & Goroshit M. (2018). General and life-domain procrastination in highly educated adults in Israel. *Frontiers in Psychology, 9*, 1173. https://doi.org/10.3389/fpsyg.2018.01173

Moscaritolo, L. M. (2009). Interventional strategies to decrease nursing student anxiety in the clinical learning environment. *Journal of Nursing Education, 48*(1), 17–23. https://doi.org/10.3928/01484834-20090101-08

Ozelie, R., Janow, J., Kreutz, C., Mulry, M. K., & Penkala, A. (2015). Supervision of occupational therapy Level II Fieldwork students: Impact on and predictors of clinician productivity. *American Journal of Occupational Therapy, 69*(1), 6901260010. https://doi.org/10.5014/ajot.2015.013532

Schrager, S. (2022). Improving time management through modern-day to-do lists. *Family Practice Management, 29*(1), 1–5. https://www.aafp.org/pubs/fpm/issues/2022/0100/p5.html

Terzi, E., Isik, U., Inan, B.C., & Ustun, U. D. (2024). University students' free time management and quality of life: The mediating role of leisure satisfaction. *BMC Psychology, 12*, 239. https://doi.org/10.1186/s40359-024-01745-2

Chapter 5

Learning and Teaching Styles and Teamwork

TOPICS

- Exploring learning styles and interpersonal communication
- Understanding your own learning styles is important
- Discovering your learning and teaching styles
- Improving how you teach your clients and their support networks
- Looking at personal influence and learning styles: Being a change agent
- Understanding groups, roles, and learning styles

I'm always just jumping into the thick of things to get started. I never appreciated the people I saw as slowing things down until we worked on identifying and trying other learning styles. I still feel frustrated when I'm ready to move on a task and others are still gathering information, but at least I'm more understanding about their behavior. It has helped in the clinic. I've learned to provide more information to some clients, even though I may feel as though they just need to stop talking and get moving. I'm still impatient, but I understand now.

—PAT, occupational therapy student finishing his last Level II fieldwork assignment

Exploring Learning Styles and Interpersonal Communication

One can look in many ways at learning styles and the influence they have on our learning, teaching, interactions, and ability to exercise personal influence. Some sources divide our skills by right-brain or left-brain strengths. Some simply divide our skills by our senses: visual, auditory, and kinesthetic. Others look at combinations of how we use our senses. Kolb (2014) divided learning styles into four categories:

1. **Concrete experiential learning** occurs when you encounter a new experience or situation. This type of learning happens every time you meet a new client or try to implement a new evaluation.
2. **Reflective observational learning** takes place when you reflect on an experience and consider its implications. This type of learning occurs when you debrief with your fieldwork educator and review how a client session went.
3. **Abstract conceptualization** is how you develop abstract concepts and theories based on reflection. The conclusions you draw from the client interaction and what knowledge or skills you gained from the clinical encounter are an example of abstract conceptualization.
4. **Active experimental learning** occurs when you apply theories to new situations to gain more experiences. You must continually try out what you learn. When you learn from mistakes or treatment sessions that don't go quite as planned because you actively experimented with a theory of what might work with a client, you are engaging in active experimental learning.

Kolb argued that we must learn to use all four areas to complete the reflective process during experiential learning activities. As occupational therapy practitioners, we need these skills to adjust our interventions to the learning styles of our clients because the trauma of what brings them to us may reduce their flexibility to adjust their learning styles. You also need to understand learning styles so you can articulate where you may be struggling to your fieldwork educator who might then be able to adjust to help you.

Gardner (2024) broke down learning into seven intelligences that affect how we learn, store, and use what we know:

1. **Body/kinesthetic intelligence** involves learning, understanding, and using information through movement.
2. **Interpersonal intelligence** includes verbal and nonverbal interactions with others, group cooperation, sensitivity to other people's emotions, and the ability to adjust personal goals to meet group goals.
3. **Intrapersonal intelligence** relates to self-awareness, including a spiritual quality, use of introspection and reflection, and the understanding of how our own emotions affect ourselves and those around us.
4. **Logical/mathematical intelligence** involves more than working with numbers—it is how we organize our environment to make rational sense of it, including inductive and deductive reasoning. It includes seeing patterns in our environment, behaviors, and reactions to those around us. It is especially important in seeing relationships, old experiences, and new situations.

5. **Music/rhythmic intelligence** refers to understanding or making sense of patterns of sound in our environment and inflections in speech, music, or other common sounds in our surroundings. Some languages depend on understanding the meanings related to pronunciation, intonation, or sound because the musical quality of pronunciation can change the meaning of the word.
6. **Verbal/linguistic intelligence** relates to the meaning of written and oral language, and being able to make sense of it in both concrete and abstract ways.
7. **Visual/spatial intelligence** refers to figure–ground and spatial relationships that are used to make meaning of our environment and to help us understand our body parts and objects in our environment. For example, we recognize shoes as different from eating utensils, and we can use guided imagery or other activities that require us to imagine rather than touch our environment.

Understanding your preferred modes of intelligence can inform the clinical education process and provide useful information for your fieldwork educator to help you leverage your multiple intelligences (Lane, 2010).

Understanding Your Own Learning Styles Is Important

You need to be a lifelong learner so you can help your clients, their circles of friends, and their caregivers to create meaningful experiences in all occupational areas. You may not always have enough time to effect changes yourself, but you can be a resource and provide people with information to assist them in their learning. They may realize the usefulness later and be able to use resources because of your recommendations. Even when the client cannot apply ideas immediately, you still can present them to meet the client's and others' learning styles.

Using various learning styles to give information can help your clients derive meaning from experiences, and help you understand their needs and offer them resources for the future. However, you must first understand your strongest learning style and the strengths and biases of that style; only then will you be able to distinguish your own window to learning—how you see the world—from how your clients view information or situations.

People often choose careers that are associated with their learning styles. You have probably chosen occupational therapy because you are fascinated by the combination of mind, body, culture, and life experiences that affect a person's choices and performance of activities. What makes something easy for some people, challenging for others, and seemingly impossible for others? Why are some clients so easy to work with, and others are so difficult? Why do some people get a "rush" from the challenge of working with the most demanding clients? The answers to these questions reflect our differences and are influenced by our learning styles.

Talk It Over With Your Fieldwork Supervisor

Discussing your learning style preferences with your fieldwork supervisor may decrease the repetition of information and increase your ability to apply suggestions immediately. Consider these questions:

- Is it easier to learn by actively doing something, or do you prefer to follow a written list of tips or steps?
- Do you need to take notes, or does taking notes interfere with your ability to listen?

Let your supervisor know how you best process and apply new information.

Discovering Your Learning and Teaching Styles

Help your fieldwork supervisor give you more meaningful feedback and instruction by completing the exercises in this and other chapters. You don't need to share the exercises with your supervisor, but you will learn information as well as techniques for organizing your work and resources that will make you more successful in fieldwork and beyond. In addition to the exercises, you can find sources online that help you examine your own learning styles, learn the most effective teaching styles for communicating the ways in which others learn and process information, and understand those ways. Some websites include quizzes that can help clarify learning differences for you.

To discover your own learning styles, consider these questions:

- How would you describe yourself based on your favorite learning styles?
- Do you use a mixture of learning styles?
- Which learning styles are most comfortable?
- Which ones raise your anxiety when trying to process information?

Your clients may lack the flexibility to use multiple learning styles because of anxiety about needing therapy and meeting a new therapy provider. See Exhibit 5.1 for an example of a personal assessment of learning styles. Then complete Exercise 5.1 to help you describe your learning needs and style to your fieldwork supervisors.

EXHIBIT 5.1. Personal Assessment of Learning Styles and Comfort Levels

Listening/Auditory (Percentage of Comfort With This Style)	Seeing/Visual (Percentage of Comfort With This Style)	Touching/ Kinesthetic (Percentage of Comfort With This Style)	Total (Must Equal 100%)
(20%) I listen well, but I don't always retain what I have heard until I write it down. It seems to be a more immediate type of learning for me. Mnemonics are lost on me unless there is movement involved.	(35%) Seeing things works well for me. I have good observation skills. I seem to catch onto things being told to me if I have them in writing to follow at the same time. Once I've written something, it's like I can see the writing. And I don't often have to go back to my notes.	(45%) The saying, "Getting a feel for how to do something" really seems to pertain to me. It's as though I have better memory when my muscles and movement are involved. I can look at and handle something and usually understand it, even make a pattern to replicate it.	(100%) Seems that observing, writing my own notes, and then doing something come together for my easiest learning. It's reinforced when I go over my notes with someone. Maybe that's why I like study groups.

Exercise 5.1. How Would You Describe the Percentages of Each Learning Style You Are Most Comfortable Using?

In each column, briefly describe how the learning style fits you and indicate, using a percentage, how comfortable you feel using that learning style. Then total the percentages for Columns 1–3.

Listening/Auditory	Seeing/Visual	Touching/ Kinesthetic	Total
______%	______%	______%	______%

> *I wish I had a camera one day when we experimented with learning styles in class. The groups of students—with one student playing a client with a bad back—were to teach each other how to pick up a pencil from the floor. The "active and concrete experience" people were done before I finished the instructions. Twenty minutes later, the "abstract conceptual" still wanted more specific client information, and the "reflective observation" people were distracted, watching the problems that were occurring in other groups. It was a true moment of insight for some students who had never realized that their styles of approaching a learning situation could be so different.*
>
> *As therapists, we have the responsibility to flex our teaching to meet the clients' needs, not the other way around. The more we understand about ourselves, the better we can use our skills therapeutically.*
>
> —BONNIE (co-author of this book)
> on my experience as an occupational therapy professor

One can divide or quantify intelligence in other ways. The application of the different intelligences may vary according to the task on which one is focused. Patterns of behavior may result in one losing flexibility in an area that isn't dysfunctional, just unused, like muscles that haven't been exercised for a while. Frustration, both yours and the client's, is common when something doesn't make sense to you in your primary learning style.

How would you apply your skills or focus on something based on the seven intelligences (Gardner, 2024) discussed earlier? Complete Exercise 5.2 to find out.

Exercise 5.2. Applying Gardner's Seven Intelligences

Use examples of your own activities or those you might perform when providing occupational therapy and place them next to the primary type of intelligence needed to perform that activity. Do your personal preferences fall into certain categories of strengths? Are there activities that you could perform that would "exercise" the other areas?

Gardner's Intelligences	Your Examples
Body/kinesthetic	
Interpersonal	
Intrapersonal	
Logical/mathematical	
Music/rhythmic	
Verbal/linguistic	
Visual/spatial	

Source. Types of intelligences from Gardner (2024).

Improving How You Teach Your Clients and Their Support Networks

Understanding learning styles can help you during fieldwork and as a clinician when you are teaching or educating clients and their support networks. Consider the following examples:

- You hand a client an information sheet. You may need to provide examples, describe actions, or ask the client to demonstrate while you observe how the information is used.
  Solution: Always try to provide your client with written, oral, and kinesthetic information. When receiving information from others, request your own best ways to receive information. Remember that too much information can be confusing.
- You or someone else demonstrates something. The client may need an instructional handout to follow and reinforce information while it is being demonstrated, or they may prefer to write the information down themselves to recall and apply it.
  Solution: Ask before you demonstrate. Allow your client to choose their own technique to help them retain information. As the occupational therapy practitioner, you and not the client should demonstrate the greatest amount of flexibility in transmitting information and a variety of learning styles to your client.
- Someone asks you or a client to do something without adequate explanation ("adequate" from the client's or your perspective). The client or you may be immobilized because there is not enough information from the client's or your perspective.
  Solution: It's up to you. What problems can arise in this situation? What possible behaviors would show in the givers and receivers of instruction? How would you respond if you were the person who thinks they have given full instruction? How would you respond as the receiver of instruction you don't understand?

Consider who may have a tendency to just jump into doing something. Who might want more information before taking action? Understanding how these needs in clients and their support networks can be met can help them functionally and consistently act on your instructions. Refining your ability to relate to others' learning and teaching styles will also help you work in interprofessional teams.

One technique that can help understand and educate clients involves clustering them into four general, broad categories describing their behavior:

1. **Relationships and harmonizing.** People with this focus tend to maintain harmony in groups; however, in excess, they can seek "peace at any price," excluding failure to take action.
2. **Reflective activities and theory building.** People with this focus tend to look for patterns and analyze behaviors. They also work to maintain and preserve the status quo and avoid change.
3. **Pragmatic elements.** People with this focus like to get things done now and to organize and direct. In excess, they might appear insensitive to others' feelings and appear impulsive; in some situations, they may push the limits of acceptable behavior.

4. **Interpreting feelings, critical analysis, and achieving perfection.** People with this focus like to understand a situation and care for people's feelings. In excess, they can appear slow to take action, be overly critical, and be insensitive to personal privacy.

No one person falls into only one category, but the clusters can help people clarify misunderstandings. Each category has functional qualities. When a person is operating under stress or is experiencing information overload or emotional interference, the behaviors can be exhibited in excess and be dysfunctional. Some people, especially clients in distress, operate in dysfunctional excess most of the time.

Looking at Personal Influence and Learning Styles: Being a Change Agent

Continue to develop flexibility in your learning and teaching styles. This makes it easier for a wide variety of people to understand you. Because of stress of injury, disease, or disability causing unfamiliar changes in their life, your client will need more flexibility from you, but also will need to understand the information you are providing. Their stress means that you, the clinician, *must* be the one who provides flexibility. You cannot expect the client to adapt to your style.

How can you be a change agent for your client and your profession? Tables 5.1 through 5.4 help you identify behaviors, responses, and helpful hints when dealing with someone whose style differs from yours. These four tables specifically focus on the four categories describing people's behavior that were listed earlier in the section "Improving How You Teach Your Clients and Their Support Networks" and are just one method of interpreting behaviors and are not the only ones!

We all go into "excess" at times. Use the tips offered in Table 5.5 to inform others of the best ways to approach you and what to do when you need to communicate feedback to others or receive feedback. Become as aware of your "excesses"—or stress—as you are of observing clients' excesses. Table 5.6 illustrates the interactive effect of different styles, including when people are in excess.

Understanding Groups, Roles, and Learning Styles

The roles that people play in groups are often related to their ways of learning and gaining control of situations or their environment. Our first experiences as members of a group occur in our families. Understanding the roles you tend to play will help you improve, contribute to groups, recognize the roles others play, and promote a more productive group experience. We are not always aware of the roles we play. Recognizing your role in the group process is another learning process requiring critical self-assessment!

TABLE 5.1. Summary Relationships and Harmonizing Category

This table shows the strengths and weaknesses of people whose interactive styles are focused on building relationships and on harmony.

Basic orientation: You have to be sensitive to, and harmonious with, the needs and wants of others. By adapting yourself to others and filling their needs first, you can then have your needs and wants filled.

Personal goal: To be seen as likable and popular

Quote reflecting this category: "Peace at any price."

Productive Use of Strengths (Productive Style)	Excessive Use of Strengths Under Stress (Stress Style)	Excessive Use of Strengths in Conflict or Disagreement (Fight Style)	Strength/ Weakness Irony Productive → Excessive
• Uses social skills and personal charm to cope with reality in the world • Emphasizes adapting and fitting in with others • Has a youthful manner, jokes, and is not serious • Shows social sensitivity to others' needs; has an underlying philosophy of "if you want to get along, find out what others need, and see that they get it"	• Is oversolicitous • Becomes childlike and is fond of horseplay • Tends to look foolish at times • Can lose sense of own identity • Becomes ambivalent, too flexible	• Overcompromises and gives the appearance of going along • Avoids confrontations even if they do not believe others are right • Keeps harmony at all costs	Flexible → Inconsistent Experimenting → Aimless Youthful → Childlike Enthusiastic → Agitated Tactful → Overagreeable Adaptable → Lacks conviction Socially skillful → Manipulative Negotiating → Overcompromising Animated → Melodramatic Inspiring → Unrealistic Sociable → Unable to be alone Solicitous → Fawning Entertaining → Foolish Complimentary → Flattering

TABLE 5.2. Summary of the Category Focusing on Reflective Activities and Theory Building

This table shows the strengths and weaknesses of people whose interactive styles are focused on reflecting and building theories about how things happen.

Basic orientation: You have to preserve what you have and use existing resources to build the future on the past in a careful and rational way.

Personal goal: To be seen as objective and rational

Quote reflecting this category: "Look before you leap."

Productive Use of Strengths (Productive Style)	Excessive Use of Strengths Under Stress (Stress Style)	Excessive Use of Strengths in Conflict or Disagreement (Fight Style)	Strength/ Weakness Irony Productive → Excessive
• Relies strongly on logic, facts, and systems • Often weighs all alternatives to eliminate risk • Has need for predictability, no surprises • Maximizes use of procedures and policies • Must prove practicality of change to convince them of need of change • Has an underlying philosophy of "you have to preserve what you have and build the future on the past"	• Develops "analysis paralysis" (i.e., freezes under pressure) • Holds onto old ways and things in the face of necessity for change	• Amasses large number of facts to support their case, then expects others to see their viewpoint • Becomes stubborn, cold, or withdrawn • Disengages from the situation and waits for others to come to them	Tenacious → Cannot let go Practical → Uncreative Economical → Stingy Reserved → Unfriendly Factual → Data-bound Steadfast → Stubborn Thorough → Elaborate Methodical → Plodding Detail-oriented → Nit-picking Analytical → Critical Composed → Unfeeling Cautious → Non–risk-taking Realistic → Unimaginative Logical → Overstructured

TABLE 5.3. Summary of the Category Focusing on Pragmatic Elements

This table shows the strengths and weaknesses of people whose interactive styles are focused on a pragmatic view of life and a direction toward achieving what they believe are very practical goals.

Basic orientation: If you want things to happen, you've got to make them happen and convince people to trust your competence. You cannot wait for things to come to you.

Personal goal: To be seen as active and competent

Quote reflecting this category: "Go for it!"

Productive Use of Strengths (Productive Style)	Excessive Use of Strengths Under Stress (Stress Style)	Excessive Use of Strengths in Conflict or Disagreement (Fight Style)	Strength/ Weakness Irony Productive → Excessive
• Likes to take charge, command, and control • Is quick to act or take a risk • Likes challenge, a chance to master a difficulty • Seeks variety and novelty • Prefers to direct and coordinate the work of others • Seizes an opportunity when they see it • Has an underlying philosophy of "if you want things to happen, you must make them happen"	• Becomes manipulative • Becomes impulsive • Likes new things for the sake of newness; abandons the old even if still useful • Takes opportunity and autonomy away from others	• Tends to openly demand their own way • Quick to defend their position • Is combat ready and becomes coercive • Can fight for their rights to the bitter end	Controlling → Domineering Quick to act → Impulsive Self-confident → Arrogant Seeks change → Drops old ways Is persuasive → Distorts Forceful → Coercive Competitive → Contentious Risk taker → Gambler Persists → Relentless Urgency → Impatience Enterprising → Opportunistic Self-starter → Overexerts Imaginative → Unrealistic

TABLE 5.4. Summary of the Category Focusing on Interpreting Feelings, Critical Analysis, and Achieving Perfection

This table shows the strengths and weaknesses of people whose interactive styles focus on interpreting other people's feelings with the goal of making things as perfect as possible.

Basic orientation: By being responsive to people, pursuing excellence, and following your ideals, your conscientiousness will be appreciated, and good things will come to you.

Personal goal: To be seen as a responsive and worthy person

Quote reflecting this category: "If it's worth doing, it's worth doing well."

Productive Use of Strengths (Productive Style)	Excessive Use of Strengths Under Stress (Stress Style)	Excessive Use of Strengths in Conflict or Disagreement (Fight Style)	Strength/ Weakness Irony Productive → Excessive
• Has very high standards for self and others • Admires and supports others' accomplishments • Has great trust and belief in other people • Is eager to respond when help is solicited • Is very idealistic • Believes that if they are conscientious and prove their worth, they will be rewarded without asking	• Becomes overly trusting and gullible • Pushes the style so hard it becomes deferential • Is vulnerable to disappointment when goals are high • Is easily disillusioned and disappointed in people • Suffers from loss of perspective	• Assumes the blame • Becomes unsure and solicits help; becomes dependent • Is perceived by others as being a "soft touch" • Gives in rather than fights and causes trouble	Accepting → Indulgent Cooperative → Easily influenced Thoughtful → Self-denying Idealistic → Impractical Modest → Self-deprecating Courteous → Deferential Optimistic → Unrealistic Trusting → Gullible Feeling → Sentimental Loyal → Obligated Helpful → Paternal/maternal Receptive → Passive Responsive → Overcommitted Seeks excellence → Seeks perfectionism

TABLE 5.5. Aids to Giving and Receiving Feedback Related to Learning and "Receiving" Styles

When Category 1 Style (Focus on Relationships and Harmonizing) Is Operating in Excess	**When Category 2 Style (Focus on Reflective Activities and Theory Building) Is Operating in Excess**	**When Category 3 Style (Focus on Pragmatic Elements) Is Operating in Excess**	**When Category 4 Style (Focus on Interpreting Feelings, Critical Analysis, and Achieving Perfection) Is Operating in Excess**
Pace and approach: • Be friendly and informal; socialize *first* before serious business. • Give encouragement. • Use humorous appeals.	*Pace and approach:* • Proceed in two stages. • Give time to reflect and opportunity for the person to analyze your information. • Allow for cool-off time.	*Pace and approach:* • Respond quickly. • Hear the person out and give them a chance to talk. • Reflect understanding (i.e., use active listening).	*Pace and approach:* • Be accessible, collaborate, and spend additional time. • Provide support, encouragement, and reassurance. • Appeal to ideals, principles, excellence, and sense of fairness.
Data needed:	**Data needed:**	**Data needed:**	**Data needed:**
• Let the person know you are pleased. • Show how the person fits in or belongs. • Reassure the person that they are liked by you or others.	• Provide details; use facts, data, and policies. • Tie new things to old. • Get some additional facts that the person will trust.	• Offer solutions; don't bring up new problems. • Suggest alternatives or options for viewing the problem. • Clarify your own limitations.	• Acknowledge value of intent, even if the consequences weren't as desired. • Affirm the person's worth. • Offer concrete and specific assistance.

(Continued)

TABLE 5.5. Aids to Giving and Receiving Feedback Related to Learning and "Receiving" Styles *(Cont.)*

Process:	**Process:**	**Process:**	**Process:**
• State you want to hear the person's opinion or preferences even though they may be different from yours.	• Be calm and unemotional, lower tension, and minimize emotional content. This may mean giving yourself a cooling-off period.	• Speak firmly, assert yourself, avoid "iffy" statements, and don't submit information in questions (e.g., "Here is a possibility" rather than "Could it be?")	• Show concern.
• Be willing to try for a compromise.	• Be willing to take or offer to do some work aspect, particularly related to data gathering.	• Respect the person's autonomy.	• Be team oriented and encourage mutual goal setting.
Miscellaneous:	**Miscellaneous:**	**Miscellaneous:**	**Miscellaneous:**
• Allow for "saving face."	• Discuss the criteria desired to evaluate the problem.	• Recognize the person's skills or competencies.	• Suggest some way the person can improve or "make up" for the problem.
• Provide an opportunity for the person in the spotlight to be prepared to be appreciated.	• Come to any meeting with data.	• Appreciate the person's initiative.	• Don't prod, which can be interpreted as nagging.

TABLE 5.6. Styles Interacting in Excess: The Interactive Effect of Different Styles

Find Your Style; Compare Your Responses in Stress to the Perception of Others	**These People Experience a Focus on:** Relationships and Harmonizing (Category 1)	Reflective Activities and Theory Building (Category 2)	Pragmatic Elements (Category 3)	Interpreting Feelings, Critical Analysis, and Achieving Perfection (Category 4)
	When These People Are in Excess:			
Category 1: Relationships and harmonizing	You fake me out too often, make me feel like I've been conned and uneasy with all the bull.	You are too people oriented, not practical enough.	You are too tricky, too solicitous.	You bend too much, can't be trusted.
		You joke around too much and disregard the rules.	You are a hard nut to figure out.	You are without principles, not serious enough, and not involved enough.
Category 2: Reflective, activities and theory building	You are too serious, too rigid and unbending.	You are locked into only one set of data.	You are too slow to react, bogged down with details, overly cautious.	You are too cautious and too tied down to ritual, procedure, and so on.
	You don't have enough real regard for people's feelings.		You curb what I want to do.	You are not feeling or caring enough about people.
				You are too withdrawn, unfeeling.
Category 3: Pragmatic elements	You are not heedful enough of people's reactions and are too locked into your own point of view.	You are too impulsive, too emotional, and possibly dangerous.	You are too feisty, too impulsive.	You are overbearing, ruthless, unwilling to learn, unprincipled, and overly demanding.

(Continued)

TABLE 5.6. Styles Interacting in Excess: The Interactive Effect of Different Styles *(Cont.)*

Find Your Style; Compare Your Responses in Stress to the Perception of Others	These People Experience a Focus on:			
	Relationships and Harmonizing (Category 1)	**Reflective Activities and Theory Building (Category 2)**	**Pragmatic Elements (Category 3)**	**Interpreting Feelings, Critical Analysis, and Achieving Perfection (Category 4)**
	You don't tune in enough to others.	You disregard costs and practical issues.	You go beyond the limits too often. I can't control you.	You are never satisfied. You make me feel inadequate.
Category 4: Interpreting feelings, critical analysis, achieving perfection	You are too serious, too pious, and too critical.	You are too emotional and not objective enough. You need to be more consistent and practical.	You are too needy, not action-oriented enough, too critical, and too soft. You have your head too much in the clouds.	You make me feel guilty, misunderstand me, disappoint me, and don't trust me.

Group Roles

Group roles fall into three general categories: (1) roles that enhance the learning process, (2) roles that focus on specific tasks that are group centered, and (3) roles that can negatively affect a group.

Roles that enhance the learning process

Roles that enhance the learning process are group centered or team centered and focus on building and maintaining group goals. These roles include the following:

- **The enhancer:** This role praises, agrees with, and accepts the contributions of others. They indicate warmth and solidarity in their attitude toward the other group members; offer commendation and praise; and indicate understanding and acceptance of other points of view, ideas, and suggestions.
- **The harmonizer:** This role mediates the differences among other members, attempting to reconcile differences and relieve tension in conflicts through joking or calming behaviors.

- **The compromiser:** This role operates as a participant in conflict in which their own positions are involved. They may offer compromise by yielding status, admitting error, disciplining themselves to maintain group harmony, or offering suggestions to bring the group to consensus or agreement.
- **The gatekeeper and expeditor:** This role facilitates the participation of others and proposes regulation of the flow of comments to allow turn-taking to balance the discussion in a timely manner.
- **The standard setter:** This role expresses, paraphrases, and helps members maintain standards to which the group has agreed related to discussion or behaviors intended to move the group toward completion of its purpose.
- **The observer and commentator:** This role keeps records, often acts as secretary, maintains a history of the group actions, provides consistency, and acts as a way for the group to evaluate its progress.
- **The follower:** This role goes along with the movement of the group. They may appear passive at times or serve as the audience to the discussion and decisions. In the best of all possible group interactions, the follower often changes roles with other group members, flowing between leadership and followers to promote the best use of skills and talents of the group so that it may achieve its objectives or purpose.

Roles that focus on specific tasks that are group centered

Group roles exist that focus on specific group-centered tasks and activate members of the group to produce positive results. The following are descriptions of each role:

- **The information seeker:** This role asks for clarification of suggestions made regarding their factual adequacy and focuses on authoritative information and facts pertaining to the group task.
- **The opinion seeker:** This role asks for clarification of the values pertinent to what the group is understanding or how the group values a suggestion or an alternative approach, rather than asking for factual data.
- **The information giver:** This role offers facts or generalizations that are authoritative or relate to the information giver's own experience when it is pertinent to the group problem.
- **The opinion giver:** This role states their belief or opinion pertinent to a suggestion made or offers alternative suggestions, emphasizing their proposal of what should become the group's view. They may ignore relevant facts or information to focus on their own suggestions.
- **The elaborator:** This role spells out suggestions in terms of examples or relevant meanings to the group members. They offer rationales for suggestions and provide ideas related to how an idea or suggestion would work out if adopted by the group.
- **The coordinator:** This role shows or clarifies the relationships among various ideas or suggestions, tries to connect ideas or suggestions, and coordinates the activities of members or subgroups.

- **The orienter:** This role defines the position of the group relative to what is currently happening. If the group has defined its goals or direction, this role raises questions to redirect discussion when the group appears to be deviating from its goals.
- **The energizer:** This role prods the group into action or decisions and keeps the group stimulated to achieve its goals and remain focused on the task at hand.
- **The procedural technician:** This role performs routine group tasks and expedites the group process by distributing materials, arranging chairs, cleaning up after the group, and performing other tasks that help the group continue toward its goals.
- **The recorder:** This role keeps the written record or history of the group decisions and tasks and maintains the group memory.

Roles that can negatively affect a group

Roles that can negatively affect group and interpersonal interactions tend to be self-serving or self-focused rather than group focused. People who assume distractor roles are not necessarily negative. These roles are often the result of poorly initiated group processes, such as the establishment of a group task by an authoritative leader who expects the group to come to the leader's preconceived conclusion, dictates inappropriate goals for the group to achieve, sees members as lacking the experience to function in groups, or brings groups together without adequate definitions of their task. These group members often need to learn about each other, become familiar with the task that brings them together, and be appreciated for the contribution they can bring to the task.

It takes time and a clear purpose for group members to come together and be functional. It also takes energy to overcome experiences that developed past behaviors exhibited in negative roles. The roles include the following:

- **The aggressor:** This role works through intimidation by deflating the value of other members, taking credit for other members' work, or ridiculing the group's goals.
- **The blocker:** This role often calls themselves "the devil's advocate" and dismisses ideas with negative comments or attitude. They may try to block proposals by continually bringing up ideas that the group has already dismissed or proven to have failed or to have had adverse outcomes.
- **The recognition seeker:** This role focuses attention on themselves through boasting of personal achievements and name-dropping with the goal of increasing personal status at the expense of other group members whom they consider inferior.
- **The self-confessor, help seeker:** This role works to have the group solve their personal problems or provide forgiveness related to former personal behaviors. They seek personal problem solving rather than focusing on group tasks. They usually want group sympathy more than solutions.

Which Roles Do You Play in a Group?

Identifying your most common roles can help you understand how others respond to you (see Exercise 5.3 to identify what roles you play in a group). Work toward balancing the roles you positively play and avoid assuming negative roles. In the best group situations, members trade roles in positive ways that facilitate the group achieving its goals or completing its tasks.

Most groups have a limited time to achieve goals and then disband. The bonds that seemed so intense while working together may disappear once the task is completed. It may be important to honor and celebrate group success as part of the farewell to the completed collaborative process. Group work is dynamic and constantly changing as tasks are completed; therefore, the roles we play in the group process often change, too, because each task has its own dynamics.

Learn to monitor accurate and honest self-assessment of your roles in effective or dysfunctional group processes. We all play different roles in different tasks and with different people. Being aware of your role contributes to the group's success and completion of assigned tasks.

Exercise 5.3. Identifying Your Role in a Group

Identify roles that you might play in a group and place a check mark in Columns 2 through 5 to indicate how often you play each role. As you do this exercise, consider what factors might affect what role you play depending on the task and group members. Also, consider other factors that may influence how you interact in a group setting.

Group Roles	Never	Sometimes	Often	Always
Team centered				
Encourager				
Harmonizer				
Compromiser				
Gatekeeper, expeditor				
Standard-setter				
Observer, commentator				
Follower				
Task centered				
Information seeker				
Opinion seeker				
Information giver				
Opinion giver				
Elaborator				

Group Roles	Never	Sometimes	Often	Always
Team centered				
Coordinator				
Orienter				
Energizer				
Procedural technician				
Recorder				
Negative, self-centered				
Aggressor				
Blocker				
Recognition seeker				
Self-confessor, help seeker				

I admit to not always being an effective group member. Sometimes I've felt more like making jokes or being a blocker/distractor than working on the task. I find that happens most when I'm unclear of the purpose, feeling like the decisions have been made and the group is just for show, or feel it's unimportant work. That's when I need to consider these roles and move from blocker/distractor into something more productive, even if it is just to clarify information for myself. I can be a good clarifier for others, too. It happens to most of us at one time or another. Awareness is key to keeping it in check.

—BONNIE, occupational therapist (and co-author of this book) on my experience as a group member

Summary

In this chapter, you have explored your learning and teaching styles and their effect on interpersonal communication in your personal and professional relationships. You also have examined how learning and teaching styles can affect the questions you ask, the answers you receive, and how you interpret your environment and the information you receive. Determining how your learning and teaching styles can change or become more rigid when under stress will help you provide your fieldwork supervisors with important cues for effective communication and exchange of feedback.

Tables 5.1–5.4 provide one technique to look at behavior when one is focused on one learning style rather than working in a flexible or cooperative position to adapt the situation or communication to other learning styles. Although coworkers can flex more readily into different learning styles, clients are less likely to have flexibility because of stressors that have brought them to occupational therapy interventions.

You have reviewed group behavior based on roles you might play or people with whom you might interact. The client will also play some of these roles in the rehabilitation process. The behaviors of other people or of occupational therapy practitioners can trigger unexpected behavioral responses in clients simply because their stress limits their variety of responses and behavioral control. Identifying both positive and negative group roles can help you be an effective group member and enable you to make more effective client interventions.

References

Gardner, H. (2024). Multiple intelligences and education. In K. Aubrey and A. Riley (Eds.), *Understanding and using challenging educational theories* (3rd ed., pp. 259–280). Sage.

Kolb, D. A. (2014). *The Kolb Learning Style Inventory V3.1.* Hay Group.

Lane, I. F. (2010). Professional competencies in health sciences education: from multiple intelligences to the clinic floor. *Advances in Health Science Education, 15*, 129–146. https://doi.org/10.1007/s10459-009-9172-4

PART II.

Professional Success Strategies

Chapter 6

Professional Behaviors and Expectations

TOPICS

- The importance of professionalism
- Professional communication
- How to assess your professionalism
- Goal setting for professional behaviors
- Your actions have consequences
- Learn professionalism by observing
- Professional civility

Fieldwork educators agree that we can help any student refine their skills, enhance their knowledge, and gain the clinical exposure they need to develop into an occupational therapy practitioner. However, it's harder to teach professionalism. If students show up to the rotation with a negative attitude or inappropriate professional behaviors, we are less likely to be as supportive. All fieldwork educators expect students to arrive ready to learn and willing to put in the work, which includes pitching in to clean up and striving to work well with all team members. The worst thing I have ever heard a student say is "that's not my job" when they were asked to help a rehab technician clean the therapy gym. The entire team viewed the student's response as disrespectful to the staff member. The student came across as not being a team player willing to contribute to the overall function and efficiency of the clinic environment.

—JAMI, occupational therapist (and co-author of this book)

The Importance of Professionalism

Brené Brown (2018) shared that "living into our values means that we do more than profess our values, we practice them" (p. 32). Professionalism reflects this effort, which begins with a philosophy about your work and the value you place on it.

Purtilo et al. (2014) captured what *professionalism* means in health care:

> Education in the health professions is preparation for carrying out a lifelong commitment and for realizing a certain type of lifestyle. Identity as a health care professional carries with it expectations on the part of society, as well as privileges and responsibilities. (p. 70)

Taylor (2020) argued that it is the occupational therapy practitioner's "responsibility to manage and continually strive to fortify the therapeutic relationship" (p. 55) by carefully selecting shared personal information that is relevant to the professional relationship; witnessing the joys and benefits of therapeutic interventions; and being open, nonjudgmental, and comfortable with discussions about topics that might not fit the practitioner's personal views. She added that "the genuine therapist is one who sincerely wants and makes an effort for what is best for the client" (p. 85). Professionalism involves a focus on the client's needs and the lifestyle to which they hope to return.

Discussions about professionalism in the health care sector sometimes get bogged down in details about conduct and behaviors, but professionalism is demonstrated through actions—often what appear to be very small actions. Although one may claim to care deeply about clients and may express a desire to help them reach their potential, lack of attention to everyday behavior can derail the highest aspirations. For example, promptness in submitting reports may seem less important than "really caring about the client." It may be true that you "really care," but if reports are not submitted promptly, the client may be denied payment for future treatment sessions or inconvenienced in other ways. Proper, professional caring must be supported by accurate and appropriate documentation.

Your success as an occupational therapy practitioner is primarily determined by the level of professional behavior you practice and exhibit daily. The individual actions of every health care professional have multiple effects and influence on client outcomes, the overall effectiveness of an agency or facility, and the development of your own competence.

During fieldwork, you are presented with many opportunities to enact your own philosophy of professionalism as well as what you have learned in class. How you conduct yourself during fieldwork will affect others much more than in the classroom. For example, if you were late to class as a student, you were the one who missed information. Arriving late for fieldwork can disrupt others' work schedules and change the client's treatment delivery. You are now an important part of an interconnected system and sequence of services. What you do makes a difference to your clients and colleagues. Recognizing the effects your actions have on others is one of the responsibilities of a professional.

Professional Communication

All components of professional behavior (listed in the next section) are important, but communication is fundamental to your relationship with clients and other health care professionals. The clinical pace is fast, and part of fieldwork experience is becoming accustomed to that pace. You often have limited time to make your point and pass on important information. No one is a mind reader, and eventually, we have all received the response, "And what is your point?"

Using concise, clear, and unbiased language is one of the best ways to communicate with clients in a clinical environment. Be honest and straightforward; don't be judgmental; don't use medical jargon unnecessarily; and be mindful of potential barriers, such as language, cognitive ability, or literacy (Plourde, 2020). Clear communication—with clients, colleagues, and fieldwork supervisors alike—requires you to avoid using words, intonations, and phrases that create conflict or prevent the other person from hearing the content of what you are saying. Using high or low intonation or repetitive phrases that don't add meaning to the communication can muddle the point of your message. Or you may not realize you are using a word or phrase that has other meanings. The term doesn't mean what you think you've said if it is not correctly received by those you're communicating with. Learn by listening and observing how others respond to what you say. You may need to make adjustments.

Although imparting information is crucial, listening well is equally important. In clinical settings

> with competing distractions and the pressure of productivity and time constraints, active listening is critical in delivering client-centered care across generations and cultures. It is easy to begin to listen to a client and then find oneself drifting in thought, maybe already formulating a treatment plan or thinking about how this interaction will be documented for billing purposes . . . with time constraints, it is easy to formulate a quick rebuttal to a conversation or interrupt whoever is talking to make sure our input is received. (Plourde, 2019, p. 415)

Active listening is the process of "hearing" both the verbal and nonverbal messages—that is, the entire message—that your client, colleague, or fieldwork supervisor is communicating. You can do this by

- being present in the moment,
- pausing before answering questions,
- pausing between statements,
- observing the other person's responses to facilitate good rapport,
- asking clarifying questions,
- paraphrasing the other person's statements, and
- summarizing the discussion at the end (Plourde, 2019).

Active listening requires patience, self-awareness, and practice, but it is an important tool for effective, professional communication.

How to Assess Your Professionalism

The three exercises in this chapter are intended to assist you in assessing your professional behaviors by focusing on eight components of professional behaviors:

- dependability
- competence
- communication
- integrity
- cooperation and teamwork
- empathy and compassion
- initiative
- professional appearance.

These exercises

- serve as a quick review,
- provide examples of what is expected of students during fieldwork,
- outline specific information you can use to set professional goals,
- furnish you with self-assessment tools,
- give you ways to maximize the potential assistance of your fieldwork supervisors by providing materials for discussion about expectations and appropriate ways to express professionalism, and
- help you succeed in fieldwork and prepare for future career success.

In preparing to assess your actions that demonstrate or distract from professionalism, reflect on any previous feedback you have received—perhaps from instructors, personnel at facilities you have observed, or prior work experience. Is it time to act on things you previously let slide? Once you have reflected on previous feedback, complete Exercise 6.1 to answer the question, How professional are you? Perform a self-reflection before you begin fieldwork and every 3 to 4 weeks during fieldwork experiences. Doing so will help you track your progress, reinforce areas in which you have shown improvement, and highlight areas on which you need to focus for improvement. Ask your fieldwork supervisor to give you feedback using the same evaluation questions you have asked yourself (see Exercise 6.1). Then, compare and, if possible, discuss with your fieldwork supervisor.

Exercise 6.1. Self-Reflection: How Professional Are You?

• What type of feedback regarding your professionalism have you found most helpful? • Do you prefer to have this feedback in writing or oral communication?
• During your clinical and classroom interactions, what have you found to be helpful feedback?
• What do you believe are your principal strengths?
• What do you believe are your principal weaknesses?
• What kinds of things have you done to enhance your professionalism?
• What changes do you believe need to be made (if any) to improve your personal appearance as well as your interactions?
• How can you ask your fieldwork supervisor (current or future) to give you feedback so you can improve your professional behaviors?
• What other information might you ask your fieldwork supervisor to provide to help you improve your professional appearance, communication, or ____________________?

It's not easy to be objective about your own habits and deficiencies, but you can't change things you ignore or that no one mentions to you. Use the exercises in this chapter as a springboard for discussion, which provides your fieldwork supervisor with a structured, familiar means to give you valuable feedback before completing the required fieldwork evaluation forms. By using a system in which you undergo regular and honest self-assessment and set goals (you don't have to share the goals with others, although doing so can be helpful), you increase your ability to reflect critically on your own work, a valuable technique to achieve personal and professional goals.

Goal Setting for Professional Behaviors

Your experiences during fieldwork provide you with many opportunities to develop professional skills, attitudes, behaviors, and responses. Just as you learn to set measurable goals for your clients, use the same techniques illustrated in the exercises in this section to set measurable, attainable goals for yourself.

As you begin to set your goals, take some time to first think about relevant professional skills. How might they be defined in terms of skills you are developing as an occupational therapy practitioner? Consider these:

- **Active listening:** paying full attention and listening carefully to the speaker as well as thinking about and clarifying the meaning of the speaker's message
- **Confidentiality:** not discussing or disclosing information with anyone other than those who have an ethical or legal right to know that information; you cannot share client information with anyone not involved in direct care of the client without the client's written permission, and you must be careful that discussions about clients cannot be overheard
- **Empathy:** the ability to understand and articulate the feelings and viewpoints of others regardless of any conflict or judgment related to your own views
- **Ethical performance:** abiding by the morals and "right" conduct of the society in which one lives and the guidelines of the occupation one practices
- **Feedback:** repeating what the listener has heard to ensure you understand the intent of the speaker
- **Perceptions:** awareness through the senses and impressions one has from what they have seen or heard
- **Problem solving:** assessing a situation by
    - gathering all relevant facts,
    - considering various alternatives,
    - evaluating the alternatives,
    - choosing and implementing an alternative,
    - evaluating the result, and
    - making adjustments if necessary to improve the outcome.

Use Exercise 6.2 to rate how well you are doing with different elements of professionalism and to set goals for addressing areas that need more work.

Exercise 6.2. Assessing Your Professionalism

Behavioral Goals, by Category	**Comments and Self-Assessment** Rate each behavior on the following 10-point scale: 1 (*rarely, less than 40% of the time*) 2 (*occasionally, 50%–69% of the time*) 3 (*frequently, 70%–94% of the time*) 4 (*consistently, 95%–100% of the time*)
Dependability	
Arrives on time at clinical setting	
Notifies fieldwork supervisor before start time if going to be late or absent	
Arrives on time for appointments and meetings	
Completes paperwork and documentation on time	
Follows through on treatment planning and assignments	
Dependability overall average score	
Competence	
Reviews knowledge and skills regarding clinical tasks	
Interviews clients appropriately to obtain necessary information	
Demonstrates awareness of own limitations and asks for assistance when needed	
Takes appropriate precautions to ensure safety, comfort, and rights of clients	
Demonstrates flexibility and willingness to accept changing conditions and assignments and adapts to those changes	
Prepares for changes and alternatives and shows flexibility in planning	
Locates evidence-based support for choices in treatment planning	
Competence overall average score	
Communication	
Uses a tone of voice that communicates professional confidence to clients and peers	

Shares perceptions and opinions clearly and concisely using nonjudgmental language	
Uses a level of language that is appropriate for the listener	
Avoids slang and expressions that might confuse or offend the listener	
Uses feedback effectively to check the listener's understanding	
Establishes and maintains appropriate boundaries with clients	
Communication overall average score	
Integrity	
Performs duties ethically at all times	
Respects and maintains confidentiality	
Accepts responsibility for own actions without making excuses or blaming others	
Admits mistakes and is able to take suggested corrective actions	
Values and cares for equipment and resources of the facility and wipes or sanitizes equipment when needed	
Acts with honesty and integrity	
Integrity overall average score	
Cooperation and teamwork	
Makes positive contributions to the team process	
Accepts group decisions even when personal opinion differs from the group decision	
Focuses on collaborative team goals and not on individual differences	
Gives credit to those who deserve it	
Completes own share of the work and offers to do more when needed to meet group goals	

Keeps equipment and supplies in good condition and returns them to original location, so they are quickly available for the next person needing them	
Clearly communicates information peers need so they can effectively complete their work	
Cooperation and teamwork overall average score	
Empathy and compassion	
Respects rights, opinions, and feelings of clients and coworkers	
Provides assistance, treatment, and/or services to clients and peers without personal bias or prejudice	
Listens actively to learn the feelings and needs of clients and coworkers	
Avoids demonstrating personal emotions that might interfere with therapy or client services	
Empathy and compassion overall average score	
Initiative	
Starts projects, evaluations, occupational therapy interventions, and other services without being told	
Plans, organizes, and prepares for assessments and occupational therapy interventions to maximize the time scheduled with clients	
Independently seeks information and answers to questions and formulates possible answers before asking for assistance from supervisors	
Concentrates on fieldwork when at the facility; after completing a task, looks or asks for work related to fieldwork learning experiences	
Recognizes that reading and preparation must be done outside the fieldwork setting; just as in classes, there is homework	

Researches client referrals, diagnoses, and/or intervention needs to gain a better understanding of conditions and the appropriate occupational therapy interventions	
Accepts feedback from supervisors and applies it appropriately	
Initiative overall average score	
Professional appearance	
Wears clothing that is always clean and appropriate to the agency and the work to be done (clinical attire never includes bare midriffs or other revealing clothing like skintight pants or low necklines) and avoids wearing clothing that can separate during client treatment	
Practices safety and respect for others by avoiding dangling jewelry; loose, long hair; strong fragrances; extreme fashion trends, or revealing clothing (these are *safety* issues, not fashion critiques)	
Practices good personal hygiene	
Uses appropriate body posture and facial expressions that send reassuring messages to clients (i.e., drops attitudes before working with clients!)	
Professional appearance overall average score	

Your Actions Have Consequences

Actions have both positive and negative consequences. Exercise 6.3 is designed to help you understand the consequences actions may have. Apply this exercise to other experiences.

Exercise 6.3. Considering the Consequences of Your Actions

Looking at the four situations described in this exercise, think about each and consider these questions:

- What are the possible positive outcomes?
- What are the possible negative outcomes?
- What additional information might be helpful in this scenario?
- Does this scenario involve student–therapist and/or client safety?

Then consider possible solutions from the points of view of clients, colleagues, and the facility and administration.

Situation 1. A student is scheduled to work at a rehabilitation hospital until 5 p.m. but does not return from lunch because they need to locate a new place to live. The student considers this an emergency and does not call their supervisor.

Possible consequences or solutions:

Situation 2. A student leaves a client unattended in the treatment area to go in search of equipment.

Possible consequences or solutions:

Situation 3. A student writes a note of appreciation to their supervisor for help in achieving a goal.

Possible consequences or solutions:

Situation 4. A student decides that personal expression is an individual right and wears eyebrow and nose rings when scheduled to work with a confused older client at a senior community center.

Possible consequences or solutions:

Talk It Over With Your Fieldwork Supervisor

Planning ahead enables you to make appropriate decisions more quickly when you experience stress. In the following five situations, suggest appropriate actions to handle each situation:

1. You become ill at the facility. What do you do, and who needs to know?
2. You have an ill child and got 2 hours of sleep the night before an early morning staff meeting. You arrive late, and the department head comments in front of everyone about your lack of punctuality. What do you do or say?
3. You are assigned to work with a client who has a diagnosis you are unfamiliar with. What do you do or say?
4. Some clients have lifestyles you find unacceptable or objectionable because of your religious beliefs or bad experiences with "people like them." With whom do you discuss these issues? What do you say and how could you phrase your concerns professionally?
5. No one clearly explains all the policies, and you unknowingly violate an important one. With whom do you discuss this issue? What do you say, and how can you phrase your concern professionally?

Now, discuss your responses with your supervisor. Are you in agreement? Does your supervisor suggest solutions that are common to or the policy of your fieldwork facility?

Learn Professionalism by Observing

One of the best ways to hone your professionalism skills is through observation. Observation is not a passive activity. It requires maintaining vigilance and looking for small behavioral observations and subtle words, movements, and body language. Use Exercise 6.4 to guide your observations of professionalism.

Exercise 6.4. Learn Professionalism by Observing

Observe the work and behaviors of the clinicians at your fieldwork facilities. Look for a role model whom you believe exemplifies professionalism.

- Briefly describe the behavior demonstrated by the role model.

• What appears to be their guiding professional values?
• What are the positive effects of this person's attitude and work?

Professional Civility

It is unprofessional to gossip, ignore your fieldwork site's dress code, be late, or fail to do your share of the work; however, it is uncivil to tell offensive jokes, use derogatory language, make demeaning comments, or use certain facial expressions (e.g., eyerolling). Professional civility requires both professionalism and civility. *Civility* is "behavior that shows respect toward another person, makes that person feel valued, and contributes to mutual respect, effective communication, and team collaboration" (Lower, 2012, para. 4). Professional civility reflects the core values and ethical principles of the AOTA Code of Ethics (American Occupational Therapy Association, 2020), which require interactions between occupational therapy practitioners and their clients, colleagues, students, and fieldwork supervisors to be fair and respectful.

During your fieldwork experience, you will interact with people who have different points of view, values, beliefs, choices, heritages, and so forth. Discretion, intelligent reflection, respectful and moderate communication, and integrity in decision making will go a long way in ensuring you are conducting yourself in a civil, professional manner (Kennell, 2024). Conducting yourself in this way demonstrates to your clients, colleagues, and fieldwork supervisor that you are a thoughtful, effective fieldwork student who takes their professional role seriously. It also prepares you for your future career—you will have many opportunities to practice professional civility!

Summary

Becoming a professional is an evolutionary process. One does not wake up one morning after spending years in college and 6-plus months on clinical fieldwork assignments and become a professional. The process of becoming fully qualified as an occupational therapy practitioner requires self-awareness as well as the desire to grow and make changes. The tools in this chapter are offered to support your efforts at becoming exhibiting professionalism during fieldwork and beyond.

References

Brown, B. (2018). *Dare to lead: Brave work. Tough conversations. Whole hearts.* Random House.

Kennell, B. K. (2024). Professional civility. In B. K. Kennel & B. S. Howard (Eds.), *Everyday ethics & occupational therapy* (pp. 331–339). AOTA Press.

Lower, J. (2012). Civility starts with you. *American Nurse.* https://www.myamericannurse.com/civitlity-starts-with-you/

Plourde, M. A. (2019). Communicating across generations and cultures. In K. Jacobs & G. L. McCormack (Eds.), *The occupational therapy manager* (6th ed., pp. 409–418). AOTA Press.

Purtilo, R. B., Haddad, A. M., & Doherty. (2014). *Health professional and patient interaction* (8th ed.). W. B. Saunders.

Taylor, R. R. (2020). *The intentional relationship: Occupational therapy and use of self* (2nd ed.). F.A. Davis.

Chapter 7

Legal, Ethical, and Educational Issues: Why Supervision Is Required and How It Can Help You

TOPICS

- Defining *supervision:* Why you need it and what it can do for you
- Tracking your supervision need
- Defining the differences among legal, ethical, and moral issues
- Applying the Golden Rule and moral sensitivity
- Applying moral and ethical decision-making to fieldwork and clinical practice

I've had aides who were really bright and intuitively related to clients or who were in college to become therapists. There's a lot that they CAN do, but legally there are lots of things in the clinic that they MAY NOT do. Sometimes, it can be difficult when the staff is limited; aides CAN do something that really SHOULD be done, but they MAY NOT do it because of legal requirements. Those legal requirements are in place to protect the client and to require the best from our profession. We have to know the difference between "can" and "may."

—LISA, occupational therapy supervisor

This chapter explains why you, as a student, will benefit from mandatory supervision during your fieldwork education. It describes legal, ethical, moral, and educational aspects related to the supervision of students and professional staff. Role delineation pertaining to students, occupational therapy assistants, occupational therapists, and aides are discussed only briefly because the information may be updated periodically. See the American Occupational Therapy Association (AOTA, n.d.) to find the most current information on occupational therapy licensure and on state licensing agencies and their laws and regulations.

As a fieldwork student, you have unique opportunities to ask questions, visit sites where occupational therapy is practiced, and see the broad range of opportunities available to you when you become an occupational therapy practitioner. Regardless of the setting in which you plan to practice, once you pass the National Board for Certification of Occupational Therapy (NBCOT®) examination, you need to be aware of the legal and ethical issues that may surface in any occupational therapy setting.

Defining *Supervision:* Why You Need It and What It Can Do for You

Occupational therapy students must be supervised. In general terms, for students, *supervision* means that you must have someone, usually on the premises, who can provide guidance and professional advice, authorize the intervention plan you are implementing with a particular client as appropriate, and review and cosign your documentation. You can benefit from consultation and discussion with your fieldwork or clinical supervisors because, by their agreement to provide supervision to you, they are putting their license and certification on the line to provide you with instruction and opportunities for your professional growth and development.

Supervision in fieldwork can be considered a hierarchical relationship in which a more experienced practitioner intervenes to instruct and evaluate a future practitioner to enhance their performance. In this role, the occupational therapy practitioner serves as a mentor and gatekeeper for new members of the profession (Costa, 2015). As a fieldwork student, you will work under your fieldwork educator's license. This means that they are legally responsible for your behavior and the services you provide to clients. If your supervisor says, "You can't do that," it is because any potential action can have consequences for them and the client. Until you pass the certification examination, you are not a legal provider, and, thus, you require supervision regardless of your skills (i.e., this is an example of "you can, but you *may not*").

Overall, supervision is "a cooperative process . . . , a joint effort to establish, maintain, and/or elevate competence . . . based on mutual understanding between the supervisor and the supervisee about each other's education, experience, credentials, and competence" (AOTA, 2020b, p. 1). The ideal supervisory relationship promotes individual growth of both the person being supervised and the supervisor, appropriate use and development of resources, creativity, and innovation toward completing both specific client-centered goals and, frequently, less formal personal goals.

When you complete your fieldwork, depending on the state regulations, you may obtain a provisional or limited permit through a state licensing board, but you are still not a legal provider until you complete all the fieldwork requirements and pass the NBCOT certification examination. As a licensed occupational therapy practitioner gains experience, supervision varies based on the practitioner's knowledge and competency, recognized credentials of expertise, and the setting in which occupational therapy is provided. Supervision needs and requirements may not end with fieldwork but may continue throughout one's career.

The Centers for Medicare & Medicaid Services (2024) specifies five levels and their corresponding types of supervision of students required for Medicare compliance (see Table 7.1). The appropriate level of supervision—and not necessarily all five—may appear in professional guidelines related to supervision, roles, and responsibilities (e.g., AOTA's [2020a] Code of Ethics) and acts governing state practices, regulatory agencies, or reimbursement agencies that require specific levels of supervision in occupational therapy practice.

Once you have passed the NBCOT examination, you are still limited to what you *can* legally do compared with what you *may* legally be able to do. As occupational therapy assistants gain experience under the supervision of new graduate occupational therapists, they likely will face this issue. Thus, collaboration between occupational therapists and occupational therapy assistants is essential. When in doubt, the assistant needs to check with the more experienced occupational therapist, the state licensing board, or AOTA staff to clarify ethical and legal practice requirements. Defining these issues is part of your professional association, and your future ability to have a license and to practice can depend on knowing your professional legal responsibilities.

Tracking Your Supervision Need

The amount of supervision you will require as a student is based on your fieldwork supervisor's observation and decision. The development of occupational therapy skills and the level of supervision needed also relate to your competence level. Some students

TABLE 7.1. Levels and Types of Formal Supervision

Supervision Level (No.)	Description of Supervision Type	Interpretation
0	Not subject to supervision	Supervision is subject to professional interpretation based on experience of provider.
1	General supervision	Supervisor is not required to be on the premises.
2	Direct supervision	Supervisor must be on the premises.
3	Personal supervision	Supervisor must be in the same room.
4	Supervision exempt	This type usually refers only to Medicare procedures and may vary widely related depending on the agency, reimburser, state practice legislation, and professional association interpretation.

Source. Adapted from the Centers for Medicare & Medicaid Services (2024).

and occupational therapy practitioners move more quickly than others through competence levels. Because everyone develops differently, students and practitioners gain specific competencies in different time frames. Table 7.2, which is based on the developmental perspectives of grasping (i.e., taking in information) and transforming (i.e., interpreting and acting on information; Costa, 2015; Kolb, 2014), shows the levels of competence and corresponding type of supervision needed at each level. The last column is for marking the date on which the supervisor has said the student or practitioner has progressed to the next level of competence. The goal in Level II fieldwork is for you to achieve the status of either advanced beginner or competent entry-level practitioner.

TABLE 7.2. Levels of Competence Related to Clinical Skills and Need for Supervision

Level	Distinction	Guiding Principle	Type of Supervision Needed	Date Achieved
Novice Can follow basic rules	No distinctions between rules and context in which the rules are applied	Basic rules and procedures	Close	
Advanced beginner Can assess and adapt to deviations from rules and procedures	Actions dictated by rules versus actions dictated by situation	Important aspects of a situation	Close	
Competent entry-level practitioner Can assess and adapt to important aspects of a situation	Actions dictated by situation versus actions dictated by general plan	General principles	Routine	
Proficient professional Can assess and adapt to deviations from plan	Actions dictated by general plan versus actions dictated by intuition	Patterns and scenarios	General	
Expert Can assess and adapt to deviations from a pattern; can focus on critical factors	Actions and situations are synonymous	Holistic, integrated images and intuition	Minimal	Not achievable during fieldwork

Costa (2015) used levels of role performance to describe the need for supervision (see Table 7.3). This is another good way to measure how much supervision you need. Remember that supervision has two purposes: to protect the client and to promote your professional growth and development. The protection and appropriate treatment of the client cannot be compromised while you learn to become an effective clinician! Some treatment decisions are based on legal, ethical, and moral requirements. Behavior must be both legal (i.e., not against the law) and ethical (i.e., meeting the standards and values of the profession).

Defining the Differences Among Legal, Ethical, and Moral Issues

The following definitions provide a foundation for understanding the professional use of the terms *legal, ethical,* or *moral:*

- **Legal:** of or based on the law; permitted by law
- **Ethical:** of or conforming to moral standards; conforming to professional standards of behavior
- **Moral:** "made up of societal guidelines for right and wrong, relational factors, judgments made within specific contexts a d sense of duty, and one's own personal values" (Howard, 2024, p. 3).

TABLE 7.3. Levels of Role Performance

Level	Major Foci	Supervision
Entry Novice and advanced beginner	• Development of skills • Socialization in expectation of the organization, peers, and the profession • Acceptance of the responsibilities and accountability in role; relevant professional activities are expected	Personal or direct
Intermediate Practitioner	• Increased independence • Mastery of basic role functions • Ability to rescind to situations based on previous experience • Specialization if frequently initiated along with increased responsibility for collaboration with other disciplines and related organizations; participation in role; relevant professional activities are increased	General or direct
Advanced Professional and expert	• Refinement of specialized skills • Understanding of complex issues affecting role functions • Contributions to the knowledge base and growth of the profession, which result in being seen as an expert, resource person; or consultant; this expertise is recognized by others within and outside the profession through leadership mentoring, research, education, and volunteerism	General or supervision exempt

Legal behavior is regulated by laws and courts that interpret the laws, whereas groups of people usually determine ethical behavior. Although the term *legal behavior* is often used interchangeably with *moral behavior,* morality tends to be interpreted as related to how an individual lives, their ethical interpretation of groups within which they live and work, or their own life roles. *Ethics* provide a way of "examining, understanding, and applying moral principles that guide behavior and actions to address specific problems or dilemmas" (Rogers & Schill, 2021, p. 2). The clinical practice of occupational therapy is governed by all three types of behavior: legal, ethical, and moral. Ethical judgments focus on normative behavior: how professionals are expected to behave rather than descriptive statements of actions people must perform. The greatest dilemmas are those in which you must apply professional codes of ethics when faced with difficult situations with clients and colleagues.

Applying the Golden Rule and Moral Sensitivity

Encountering ethical dilemmas is to be expected. Just as occupational therapy students and practitioners need to be culturally responsive, we also must practice moral sensitivity. *Moral sensitivity* involves being aware of our own moral values and accepting other people's views on moral behavior. We then need to practice *acceptance*—even if you disagree with those behaviors or viewpoints. Further, personal, situational, and normative characteristics can create interpersonal dilemmas that can interfere with developing "the optimal therapeutic relationship" (Taylor, 2020, p. 101). Occupational therapy practitioners need to remember that they can communicate moral sensitivity in "nonverbal communication [that] provides clients with information about your thoughts and feelings that may not be directly articulated" (Taylor, 2020, p. 268). Such nonverbal communication, including body language, facial expressions, distance, muscle tone, and comfort in touching a client, can convey moral sensitivity to a client about the situations or behaviors that have resulted in the need for therapeutic intervention.

Some people ground their moral sensitivity through the Golden Rule: "Do to others as you would have them do to you" (Merriam-Webster, n.d.). Moral sensitivity is required when interpreting this rule to avoid doing what you personally would want or choose to have done but, rather, doing what you would want *if you were in that person's place*, including being a part of their culture, living situation, and life roles. Strive to choose activities and interventions based on that person's wants and needs, not based on your wants, biases, or needs.

I remember planning a group activity related to kitchen skills, introducing assistive devices and upper-extremity movement. Because Easter was near, the group decided to color Easter eggs. The eggs were even planned for use in decorations for a local event. One group member was Jewish but thought it would be fun too. I was careful and asked him away from the group to be sure, and he'd always been straightforward with me about his opinions.

The day arrived, and only the Jewish man could participate for various reasons. The decorated eggs were already promised and expected for the other event. The people planning the event had even paid for six dozen eggs and all the materials to decorate them. Yes, he and I completed the project, and he delivered the decorated eggs. Was it a meaningful activity for him? Yes, because he received some unexpected individual attention and he became proficient in using several assistive devices that were important to his goal of independent living. And no, because it was not part of his culture. He found wonderful humor in the situation and told me about Jewish traditions and celebrations as we worked together. But it could have been a disaster.

—BONNIE, occupational therapist (and co-author of this book)

Applying Moral and Ethical Decision-Making to Fieldwork and Clinical Practice

As you gain practice experience applying the AOTA (2020a) *Code of Ethics* with diverse clients, you may more easily identify moral dilemmas and work with your supervisor to understand how to address them. A hallmark of a professional association is that ethics are developed related to professional practice, but how we address ethical challenges and define *professionalism* evolves over time and varies depending on the client and situation. Ethics and conduct are, therefore, constantly being refined.

As human behaviors and awareness change over time, ethical conduct needs to be reevaluated. For example, before the digital age, many ethical issues related to client confidentiality were not even part of common practice, yet digital client records are now linked globally, and cybercrimes that were something of science fiction a little more than 30 years ago are now a very real threat. Online connections through social media are the norm rather than the exception and are an easy avenue for unethical behaviors and conduct. For example, you may be excited to share your daily fieldwork experiences as a student on social media, but what can seem like a harmless post can violate patient privacy and be considered a crime and grounds for dismissal. Criminal law protects both the client and occupational therapy practitioners, so in this instance, you may have shared your story on your social media page while operating under your fieldwork supervisor's license. With just one social media post, you've put your client's well-being and privacy, and your supervisor's license, at risk.

You will run into situations—like the real-life ones presented in Exercise 7.1—that call for personal judgment. Through this exercise, you can practice noting what you think of the situation, if you have any concerns, and what you might do to resolve the situation.

Exercise 7.1. Decision Making When Resolving Situational Issues

Situation 1. An occupational therapy practitioner is scheduled to see a client with a criminal background. In reviewing the client's history, the practitioner discovers that the client's conviction involved rape. The practitioner has been a victim of rape and feels that, despite their usual moral sensitivity toward clients, they cannot treat this client.

Is the practitioner right to refuse to treat a client in this circumstance? What would be the alternatives? Is it right for the practitioner to provide treatment when they feel that their trauma may make them less empathetic to the client's needs? What is in the best interest of the practitioner? Of the client? Write down your thoughts, concerns, and possible resolution:

____

____

____

Situation 2. An occupational therapy practitioner is scheduled to see a client who has been seriously injured in an automobile accident in which they were cited for driving under the influence of alcohol. The practitioner lost a close family member in an accident caused by a drunk driver who also was injured in the crash.

What issues must the practitioner deal with to provide quality, nonjudgemental therapy? Write down your thoughts, concerns, and possible resolution:

Situation 3. An occupational therapy practitioner is scheduled to see a client who has begun sending or bringing them letters in which the client discusses love and a desire to see the practitioner outside of the clinical situation. The practitioner is flustered but flattered and confides in you that they are considering meeting the person "just for coffee" outside work.

What would you do? The practitioner is an excellent clinician from whom you have learned a great deal. Who else besides the practitioner would you discuss this with? You know clinicians who have married former clients and have strong views (either pro or con) about this situation. What do you need to consider? Write down your thoughts, concerns, and possible resolution:

Situation 4. An older client with whom you have developed rapport confides in you that a family member frequently hits them. The client then begs you not to tell anyone because the same family member provides them with help and a place to stay. The client's only other alternative living situation would be in a skilled nursing facility, and they say, "I know I'd just die if I had to go somewhere like that."

You tell the client it is important that others involved with their treatment know this information. The client replies that if you tell anyone, they will deny they ever said it. You have noticed bruises on the client's arms and legs, but they have always been explained as resulting from bumping into things or losing balance, behavior that seems legitimate because you have seen similar events happen in the clinic.

Do you tell others involved with this client's treatment—or anyone else—knowing that the client will deny the discussion with you? If you talk with someone, to whom would you go? (Many agencies specify which people you would contact.) What are the ethical issues? What are the legal issues? Write down your thoughts, concerns, and possible resolution:

Situation 5. A client is being seen following a cerebrovascular accident. Although assigned male at birth, the client has legally changed their birth name to Sally, prefers to be referred to as a woman, and prefers the use of the pronouns she/her/hers. Sally's medical record states that she was scheduled for gender reassignment surgery when she had the stroke. Her intervention requires physical contact for muscle reeducation; however, several occupational therapy practitioners who have worked with Sally have quietly mentioned to you that they find it difficult to touch her.

You treat Sally, and she tells you how comfortable she is with you as her practitioner. She also says that she knows by their touch that other occupational therapists find her disgusting. She would like to see only you, even though you are not her routine/usual therapist.

What do you do? With whom do you discuss the client's issue and preference? Write down your thoughts, concerns, and possible resolution:

What challenges do you think you will face related to clients and situations or beliefs that differ from yours? Being aware of differences is the first step toward moral sensitivity. Consider the possible areas shown in the ethical and moral dilemma grid in Exercise 7.2. Some of these issues may be quite personal; remember, though, that awareness will make it easier for you to uncover potential biases that could affect your ability to provide the best possible therapy and interventions.

You don't have to share your personal views with your clients; however, you do have to treat each client with interventions that are not influenced by the way you feel about their views. Discussing the topics in Exercise 7.2 with another occupational therapy student or occupational therapy practitioner may be useful, though. Perhaps the most effective way to cover potentially difficult topics is through a general, rather than specific, discussion. They wouldn't be called *dilemmas* if we all agreed or if the decisions were clear cut. As you observe or encounter situations that may be particular to the sites where you do fieldwork or to your personal experiences, continue to add to the topics in Exercise 7.2.

Exercise 7.2. Untangling Ethical and Moral Dilemmas

In the blank space at the bottom of the grid, left-hand side, add topics or issues particular to your fieldwork sites or personal experiences. On the right-hand side of the grid, add your responses to the questions.

Views that often cause ethical or moral disagreements or conflicts	**Ask yourself:** • **What are my own views?** • **How might a client's views differ from mine?** • **How might a coworker's views differ from your views, and how might this difference affect client services?** • **How might a coworker's views affect the work environment?**
Spirituality or religious practices	
Sexuality or sexual orientation (to whom one is attracted, such as different sex, same sex, all sexes/pansexual)	
Gender identity (a person's internal sense of being male, female, both, neither, or somewhere along the spectrum of gender)	
Gender roles or norming (tasks considered more appropriate to one particular gender, which may be influenced by generational or cultural factors)	
The need to be independent versus dependent; interdependent roles	
Preconceived ideas and biases (we all have them; they are sometimes called "preferences")	
Socioeconomic differences (e.g., income levels, attitudes, acceptable behavior, use and sharing of money)	

Talk it Over With Your Fieldwork Supervisor

You can learn a great deal about ethical dilemmas from your fieldwork supervisor. Discuss the examples with clinicians you meet during fieldwork. Ask them about dilemmas they have faced and how they resolved them. Some dilemmas are related to the situations in which clients live, some are related to widely differing views of right or wrong, and some are about making a good argument to the insurance company to justify occupational therapy. Considering a wide variety of scenarios now will help you when faced with the actual situations and dilemmas to justify or discontinue therapy. Using AOTA's *Code of Ethics*, the goal is for each client to receive appropriate consideration for occupational therapy, to treat each client equitably, and to appropriately justify each client's need to receive occupational therapy as necessary.

Summary

This chapter focused on the legal, moral, and ethical dilemmas that are a constant part of occupational therapy practice and client interventions, and it emphasized the appropriate need for supervision. Supervision meets legal requirements and offers opportunities to discuss and share knowledge and solutions to problems you may encounter in practice. By considering—in advance—situations that could create problems, you add to your problem-solving skills, and you can better focus on the client's issues. You cannot plan for all possibilities, but thinking through them will allow you to more easily make decisions when critical incidents occur. Proactive thinking makes it easier to discuss problems and solutions that your fieldwork supervisor—and later, as a practitioner, your clinical supervisors—may need to know for their legal, ethical, and moral responsibilities to you, the clients, and the clinic.

References

American Occupational Therapy Association. (2020a). AOTA 2020 occupational therapy code of ethics. *American Journal of Occupational Therapy, 72*(Suppl. 3), 7413410005b01.

American Occupational Therapy Association. (2020b). Guidelines for supervision, roles, and responsibilities during the delivery of occupational therapy services. *American Journal of Occupational Therapy, 74*(Suppl. 3), 7413410020. https://doi.org/10.5014/ajot.2020.74S3004

American Occupational Therapy Association. (n.d.). *Career: Licensure.* https://www.aota.org/career/state-licensure

Centers for Medicare & Medicaid Services. (2024). *Medicare benefit policy manual: Chapter 15—Covered medical and other health services* (Revision No. 125320). https://www.cms.gov/regulations-and-guidance/guidance/manuals/downloads/bp102c15.pdf

Costa, D. M. (2015). *The essential guide to occupational therapy fieldwork education* (2nd ed.). AOTA Press.

Howard, B. S. (2024). Introduction: How to use this book. In B. K. Kennell & B. S. Howard (Eds.), *Everyday ethics and occupational therapy* (pp. 3–6). AOTA Press.

Kolb, D. A. (2014). *The Kolb Learning Style Inventory V3.1.* Hay Group.

Merriam-Webster. (n.d.). *Golden Rule.* In *Merriam-Webster.com dictionary.* https://www.merriam-webster.com/dictionary/golden%20rule

Rogers, B., & Schill, A. L. (2021). Ethics and *Total Worker Health*®: Constructs for ethical decision-making and competencies for professional practice. *International Journal of Environmental Research and Public Health, 18*(19), Article 10030.

Taylor, R. R. (2020). *The intentional relationship: Occupational therapy and use of self* (2nd ed.). F.A. Davis.

Chapter 8

Working as a Team Member

TOPICS

- Teams: A health care workplace reality
- Benefits of teams
- Effective teams: What makes them work?
- Joining teams at your fieldwork sites
- On the road: From novice to entry-level practitioner
- Dealing with conflict

The dysphagia program here works really well, but it took a while to get it smoothed out. I've had extensive training in dysphagia and videofluoroscopy, but the speech-language pathologists wanted it to be their area, even though I had more training. Ultimately, we worked out a protocol acceptable to both disciplines.

Now we take turns being lead therapist on videofluoroscopies, each of us focusing on specific but important areas of dysphagia evaluations and interventions. When schedules are tight, we have confidence in each other's skills to provide dysphagia evaluation and treatment. Teamwork isn't always easy, but it is very satisfying once we gain confidence in each other's contribution to the team.

—LISA, occupational therapist

Teams: A Health Care Workplace Reality

Teams are groups of people with common goals who work together to achieve those goals, and they are an essential component of every health care delivery system. There are very few professions in which an individual does not work as part of a team. The ability to work effectively as a team member is an essential job skill for health care professionals at every level because

- the specialized roles of health care professionals are most effective in providing quality client care and service when performed harmoniously by the entire health care team;
- financial challenges confronting the health care industry do not allow any redundant and unnecessary tasks performed by individuals not working in tandem;
- increased compliance and reporting requirements make teamwork essential to meet or exceed health care standards and optimize reimbursement; and
- high demands for quality care and performance exist in the health care industry given that human lives are directly affected by caregivers: Two heads *are* better than one.

You are likely to encounter two types of teams at your fieldwork sites:

1. Naturally occurring work teams comprising professionals who have worked together for a long time, such as a rehabilitation team.
2. Teams organized with finite lifespans for a specific project, such as to create client educational materials.

Benefits of Teams

The concept of *synergy* is often used to describe the results achieved by people who work together effectively. Synergy implies that the combined efforts of individuals working together cooperatively yield greater results than those working on their own. Results can be more impactful when people work together because it enables them to learn from each other to

- provide helpful mutual feedback;
- create a greater pool of knowledge and information than any one person possesses;
- give each other support when the going gets tough; and
- brainstorm to solve problems, enhance creativity, and develop innovative ideas and solutions.

Effective health care teams have great potential for increasing the quality of client care and, at the same time, improving the work environment of the team members. Here's one way to define a team:

T = Together

E = Everyone

A = Achieves

M = More.

Effective Teams: What Makes Them Work?

Effective teams share several common characteristics:

- They have shared values that the team has discussed and clarified and on which the members agree.
- They have clearly stated goals.
- They have well-defined working roles regarding the responsibilities of the members as contributors to the goals.

Further, effective teams have members who

- are committed to achieving the team's goals,
- trust and respect each other,
- value group achievement over individual recognition, and
- practice good communication skills.

Individuals who make up a team are the most important determinants of its success. Poorly functioning teams can be demoralizing because they can drain their members' energy and enthusiasm. Members and the roles they play really do make a difference. In Chapter 5's section "Understanding Groups, Roles, and Learning Styles," we learned about the various roles that individuals play in the group process, both enhancing and detracting. In Exercise 5.3 in that chapter, you identified what role you might play in a group and how often you play that role. Now review your answers to that exercise and complete Exercise 8.1 to gain insight into group functioning and how it applies to teamwork.

Exercise 8.1. Exploring Your Role in Group Functioning

• Which roles best describe your predominant behaviors in groups, both positive and negative?
• How do your customary roles influence and challenge your contributions to the teams you join?
• How might your roles or contributions in groups change or be different between Level I and Level II fieldwork?

Take advantage of the opportunities in fieldwork, particularly Level II, to observe and refine your roles in groups. Strive to make contributions that will help the teams achieve their goals. Observe the behaviors of others to create dynamic and challenging teamwork.

Joining Teams at Your Fieldwork Sites

A valuable part of the fieldwork experience is the opportunity to observe work teams and participate initially as an observer and then as an active member of the team. Use Exercise 8.2 to guide your observations and thoughts about ways to successfully join existing teams. This exercise will help you organize information about each team and prepare to join teams at your fieldwork sites. You can ask your fieldwork supervisor for their advice and tips related to effective teamwork, or you can gather information about a team through observation. Complete a practice version of this exercise based on groups you have observed in other settings or Level I fieldwork settings.

> *Co-leading groups with other disciplines was a requirement at one of my fieldwork sites. First, I observed the groups that were available, then I was to approach the group leader from another discipline about co-leading while I was on fieldwork. My fieldwork supervisor warned me that several of the staff had never agreed to a fieldwork student as a co-leader, but these would be good groups for me to observe. She didn't identify which people she was referring to.*
>
> *I completed my observations. Imagine my surprise—and that of my fieldwork supervisor—when it was leaders of the "never" groups who approached me to offer co-leader opportunities. My work on awareness of my role and influence had paid off. In student groups, I sometimes got in trouble for being the distracting "group clown," but I knew this was a professional role. I felt reinforced for knowing the appropriate roles matched to the situations—and had a wonderful experience learning new group leadership roles.*
>
> —BONITA, occupational therapy student

Exercise 8.2. Gathering Information on a Team Before Joining

Agency or site name:
Type of team (i.e., focus, disciplines, purpose):
Purpose of the team:
Team goals or priorities (i.e., how the team knows if its work is completed):
Members or disciplines represented on the team:

• What would be my responsibilities as a member of the team?
• What would I need to know to carry out my team responsibilities?
• Where could I get help if I needed it?
• What skills would I be bringing to the team?
• How could I demonstrate support of other team members?
• What else could I do to help the team produce results and achieve its goals?
• What would I be expected to prepare and bring to team meetings?
• What else would I need to do or prepare for work on this particular team?

Talk It Over With Your Fieldwork Supervisor

Be open to recommendations and help from your clinical fieldwork supervisors. What guidance can each of them offer you as a new member at their site?

On the Road: From Novice to Entry-Level Practitioner

> *My supervisor at my work site (I'd finished fieldwork and had a REAL job) knew her project team well. I was new to the team and the only member of my racial/ethnic group. She told me ahead of time:*
>
> > *While I hate to admit it of this team, some people will not initially listen to your comments because they think you don't share common experiences. Until they get to know you, we'll discuss what you need to say ahead of team meetings. Sometimes I will state what you've discussed rather than have you say it. I will always credit you, but this team has been closed to some people until now.*
>
> *She mentored me into full team membership in what could have been a difficult situation, and we succeeded beyond expectations with our project.*
>
> —DOREEN, occupational therapist

A common misconception that Level II fieldwork students have about what will be expected of them is that students new to the clinic will demonstrate expertise rather than novice clinical skills. This is not a realistic expectation, and effective clinical supervisors do not hold this view. Progressing from novice to a proficient provider is a journey that takes time, and Level II fieldwork is one of the early beginning steps. This particular level of fieldwork provides multiple opportunities to apply your academic skills, realize the differences between academic and clinical environments, and develop practical skills and competencies.

Levels of occupational therapy practitioner competence, ranging from novice to expert clinician, are illustrated in Table 7.2 (see Chapter 7) in your Level II fieldwork supervision context. A practitioner's competence spans a continuum of knowledge and expertise. A novice relies on instructors, professors, and textbook knowledge, but an expert or master clinician combines that foundational knowledge with the ability to rapidly assess situations, deal with the unexpected, and recognize patterns or trends by combining knowledge with assessment and observation (Costa, 2007). The key characteristics that differentiate experts from novices include

- assessing situations quickly and completely;
- applying a broader base of subject and situational knowledge;
- organizing knowledge in a way that is more accessible for solving problems, including evidence of effective interventions; and
- being better able to monitor their own actions and being more aware of their errors.

Working with team members who have more experience as occupational therapy practitioners will allow you to observe their actions and solicit feedback about your work. A primary means of acquiring expertise is through teams with dynamic processes, including defined purposes, techniques to share ideas without competition, and the development of cooperative rewards. In the co-authors' experience, clients show noticeably improved outcomes in interventions with effective team dynamics. Further, technology enables teams to meet, work together, and develop solutions and interventions in both face-to-face and virtual meetings. Virtual team meetings have the added benefit that team dynamics occur asynchronously because team members may be in multiple time zones and widely distributed geographic areas; teams can form in a single workplace or across the world.

The keys for successful and effective teams are having a clear team focus and goals while also acknowledging limitations in the time a team exists—from a few sessions to throughout the life of the agency (Pfeiffer, 2010; Poulton & West, 2010). Consider the questions in Exercise 8.3 in relation to your work with other members of the teams at your fieldwork sites. How do you acquire expertise on a team?

Exercise 8.3. **Acquiring Expertise Through Teamwork**

• What are the opportunities for working with and learning from others?
• If the opportunities are limited, what can I do to expand my opportunities for working with and learning from others outside the specific fieldwork site?
• How can I maximize these opportunities?
• What am I learning from discussion and observation about how the master clinicians assess situations and clients?

Dealing With Conflict

Conflict is a natural outcome when people with various experiences, individual styles of learning and working, and different approaches to problem solving are working together toward a common goal. Even among the most functional and optimally working teams, conflict occasionally occurs. Some conflicts are considered normal steps in forming effective groups, but groups do not become effective if they become mired in conflict.

Conflict among team members can be constructive when it

- helps the team bring issues to the surface so they can be resolved;
- encourages the sharing of information, opinions, and feelings related to group goals; and
- promotes team and individual growth.

Identifying Your Conflict Management Style

Individuals handle conflict differently, so it is helpful for them to recognize their conflict management style. Table 8.1 lists the five most frequently used styles. Use this table to find the style that best describes your most common approach to conflict, then complete Exercise 8.4 to identify your own conflict management style.

TABLE 8.1. Conflict Management Styles

Style	Usual Outcome for Self–Other	These Behaviors Are Demonstrated by Participants as Part of the Process
Collaborating	Win–win	• Viewing conflict as an opportunity to grow • Identifying underlying issues • Listening to others • Purposefully aiming for win–win solutions
Compromising	Partial win–partial win; sometimes viewed as partial loss–partial loss	• Listening to others • Giving up something • Splitting the difference • Developing solutions that partially satisfy everyone
Competing	Win–lose	• Defending your position • Taking charge • Seeking quick resolution • Trying to win as the goal
Accommodating	Lose–win	• Listening to others • Wanting to help others • Deferring to others • Giving up one's own needs
Avoiding	Lose–lose	• Denying a problem exists • Accepting the source of conflict • Delaying confrontation • Discouraging unpleasantness even if it would lead to conflict resolution

Exercise 8.4. Identifying Your Conflict Management Style

• What is your predominant conflict management style?
• What are your strengths in dealing with conflict?
• How might you be more effective in dealing with conflict?

Determining Which Style to Use

Collaboration is the most effective way to manage conflict. In team settings, collaborative efforts focus on finding constructive resolutions. Members work together, learn from each other, try to uncover the root causes of problems, and look for long-term and mutually supportive solutions. However, no single conflict management style works in every situation. You may disagree with your supervisor about an issue but not feel it is serious enough to pursue. In this situation, accommodation may be best. If a client or caregiver is possibly considering a dangerous situation, a win–lose solution (i.e., the competing style) may be the only way to ensure their safety. When an issue involves a breach of ethics by another person, strongly defending your stance regardless of the other person's position may be required; a compromise would not resolve the problem. Although compromise may be the better way to deal with many issues that must be resolved quickly, not everything can be resolved safely and ethically through compromise.

Remember that conflict is natural, but for it to be constructive rather than detrimental, you need to apply resolution techniques. As a proactive move, before you begin fieldwork, use the following prompts to consider situations in which conflict has occurred for you. Revisit these prompts when observing or being involved in conflict during your fieldwork experiences:

- Describe a situation in which an approach other than collaboration may be the best approach.
- Observe and describe how conflict is managed by other individuals in your fieldwork experiences.

Summary

Level I fieldwork introduces you to the environment in which you will later practice occupational therapy. Level II fieldwork gives you a chance to join a treatment team, more closely observe several treatment teams than you could in Level I fieldwork, and become a full member of a treatment team for a short period. You have probably had opportunities in class to try different participatory styles or to work in effective or dysfunctional teams. Take advantage of these unique opportunities to observe and study working teams in action, including your role and skills in contributing to the team. Working teams sometimes differ greatly from classroom or academic teams in that working teams may view the natural conflict that can develop in teams as opportunities for growth and improvement. Try to resolve conflict through collaboration. Developing strategies to increase your worth as a team member will significantly increase your value as an occupational therapy practitioner.

References

Costa, D. M. (2007). *Clinical supervision in occupational therapy: A guide for fieldwork and practice.* AOTA Press.

Pfeiffer, S. I. (2010). The problems facing multidisciplinary teams: As perceived by team members. *Psychology in Schools, 18,* 330–333. https://doi.org/10.1002/1520-6807(198107)18:3%3C330::AID-PITS2310180314%3E3.0.CO;2-Q

Poulton, B. C., & West, M. A. (2010). Effective multidisciplinary teamwork in primary health care. *Journal of Advanced Nursing, 18*(6), 918–925. https://doi.org/10.1046/j.1365-2648.1993.18060918.x

Chapter 9

Occupational Therapy Practice Settings and Therapeutic Applications

TOPIC

- Traditional, nontraditional, and emerging and/or and innovative practice settings

I'm eclectic, although I know that's a dirty word to some occupational therapists. That doesn't mean I don't know the frames of reference, but I don't find one frame of reference that fits all situations. I still have to know the frames of reference, so I know why I choose certain interventions over others, and it keeps me grounded in using appropriate practice. It even guides me in selecting appropriate evaluation tools.

I notice that I tend to favor some frames of reference over others partly due to the types of clients I see. The frames of reference help me understand why I select different things for different clients and why I think my professional practice is solidly grounded in theories. In a way, the frames of reference provide the metaphors through which I can assess the clients and on which I can base treatment. There's a big difference between just picking what seems handy and really using theories in an eclectic way.

—BONNIE, occupational therapist (and co-author of this book)
on my experience with frames of reference

The purpose of this chapter is to provide a way for you to organize your knowledge about *frames of reference,* which organize clinical occupational therapy practice through particular theoretical perspectives; learn how to apply the ones that drive clinical decision-making and client intervention strategies; and understand how those relate to particular clinical settings and the clients that they serve. Occupational therapy practitioners use frames of reference to evaluate the use of certain interventions (Kramer et al., 2023).

Complete the exercises in this chapter for each Level I and Level II fieldwork site, and then review them with your fieldwork supervisors to help you clarify how a theory is used in a specific clinic where you are doing your fieldwork. Many clinical settings will be driven by more than one frame of reference; therefore, three copies of Exercise 9.1 are included in this chapter for your use. The structure of that exercise will help you see the variety of therapeutic approaches that the occupational therapy frames of reference support and how they are founded. Make more copies as needed as the application of frames of reference is clarified through your fieldwork experiences. Consider using this process to clarify your understanding of the sites where you will work as an occupational therapy practitioner.

Because many books and journal articles are available to explain frames of reference, that idea is not explained here. Use your resources and textbooks to select possible theories for various client situations; this is one of the reasons your academic instructors often say, "Keep your textbooks to use for reference and resource materials." The goal of this chapter is to help you understand the clinical applications of frames of reference in specific settings and to provide you with a foundation for discussing them with your fieldwork supervisors.

Traditional, Nontraditional, and Emerging and/or Innovative Practice Settings

A clinic/agency or treatment setting's mission, the client referral base, funding, and available locations to provide occupational therapy interventions shape that setting. Sometimes, it can be confusing when the terms *traditional*, *nontraditional*, and *emerging and/or innovative* are applied to different settings. There are no absolute definitions of those words. Every setting works at being innovative; that is the creative part of being in the profession of occupational therapy. Innovation may occur in the activities selected for treatment sessions, in the adaptations to promote client success, in the documentation techniques, or in how occupational therapists and occupational therapy assistants share caseloads and how their partnership works smoothly in relation to the clients with whom they work.

Traditional Practice Setting

A *traditional practice setting* tends to be one that has been around for many years and usually describes positions within institutional care, such as hospitals, physical rehabilitation centers, mental health settings, and skilled nursing or convalescent centers. The designation of such settings as "traditional" may be the result of the laws and regulations governing what can be done in those settings and how services are reimbursed. Traditional practice settings tend to use the medical and rehabilitation models.

Nontraditional Practice Setting

A *nontraditional practice setting* tends to be one that has begun to provide services more recently or that uses less traditional occupational therapy services. This setting is often community based, such as home health, telehealth, or ergonomic consultations or functional capacity evaluations in work environments. Occupational therapy practitioners may work with professional organizations or associations whose members are at risk of injuries related to their profession, such as carpal tunnel injuries among workers in dentistry, or in other industries with a higher-than-average incidence of wrist, elbow, shoulder, and neck injuries. In addition, a number of businesses support occupational therapy staff positions that provide interventions at the worksite to proactively prevent injury among the employees.

Emerging and/or Innovative Practice Setting

As a nontraditional practice setting—that is, a less institutionally based one—becomes more common, it transforms into what is known as an *emerging and/or innovative practice setting* because occupational therapy practitioners have established an innovative (i.e., new) body of knowledge and shared best practices that are supported by research and documented outcomes of successful occupational therapy interventions. As practitioners document outcomes and establish more innovative practice sites, the practice setting then shifts from an innovative to an established area of occupational therapy practice. Community-based treatment settings are an example of this type of move from a nontraditional and innovative area to a more common and publicly understood area of occupational therapy provision. Examples of innovative practice areas that have shifted to more visible and common practice areas include day treatment centers for children and adults (sometimes in the same location to allow for intergenerational contact), life skills treatment in homeless shelters, and life skills programs for foster children who are within 2 years of emancipation when fewer services are available and who have a high risk of homelessness following foster care. Other examples of innovative locations that now provide more traditional occupational therapy interventions are community centers and churches as well as medical health clinics that formerly were emergency care settings but can now provide a range of routine health services. Mental health programs that were traditionally provided in residential or inpatient locations are now more common in schools and community settings, a proactive public health approach to address the social–emotional well-being of all students while decreasing stigma around mental health challenges.

Keep in mind that the terms *traditional, nontraditional,* and *emerging and/or innovative* do not refer to whether the therapy is conducted with individuals or groups. These terms may indicate how clients are referred, when or where intervention is provided, or who provides reimbursement or funding for services (e.g., medical insurance, unions that provide reimbursement, educational systems that provide reimbursement, grant-funded programs). Nontraditional services are often provided earlier using a prevention or health promotion model rather than traditional medical model interventions.

Why is it important for you, as a student, to consider the distinctions among traditional, nontraditional, and emerging and/or innovative practice settings? When you complete your Level II fieldwork, you will soon be looking for a job and entering the profession. You will be looking for a good fit with your skills, your continued development as an occupational therapy practitioner, your need for creativity, and your need for structure. There is no right or wrong choice. The setting is about your occupational fit to ensure success and further career opportunities.

Talk It Over With Your Fieldwork Supervisor

Talk with your supervisor about their perception: How is the site traditional, nontraditional, or emerging and/or innovative? Does the site have elements of each? In what ways does the site demonstrate these qualities?

Exhibit 9.1 describes how one frame of reference—neurodevelopmental treatment—might be used in a treatment setting and how you might compare the information to your own clinical setting. Be sure to spend some time using Exhibit 9.1 and discussing with your clinical supervisor the ways in which frames of reference may be used in your particular setting. Then, complete the next exercise, which consists of four copies—Exercises 9.1.1, 9.1.2, 9.1.3, and 9.1.4—to provide you with materials for different settings in which you do fieldwork.

EXHIBIT 9.1. Frames of Reference and Clinical Settings

Fieldwork Site: Outpatient Pediatrics	Frame of Reference: Acquisitional
Typical client diagnoses and reason for referral: • Any developmental delay or history of prematurity • Cerebral palsy • Down syndrome	How this frame of reference is applied with clients: • The goal of therapy using this frame of reference is to help children acquire and learn functional and developmentally appropriate behaviors and skills. • Learning is accomplished by interacting with a reinforcing environment through practice and repetition.
What would be a common goal for intervention related to this frame of reference in this particular setting? • A common goal would be teaching a child how to don a button-down shirt themself by breaking down the task into smaller steps and using positive reinforcement for each completed step.	What other influences does this frame of reference have in this particular setting? • This clinical setting has educated all members of the treatment team to use acquisitional frame of reference principles when the client is with occupational therapy, physical therapy, or speech-language pathology.

Exercise 9.1.1. **Fieldwork Sites and Frames of Reference**

Fieldwork or clinical site:	Frame(s) of reference:
Types of clients (i.e., diagnoses or reason for referral):	How this frame of reference is applied with clients:
What would be common goals for intervention related to this frame of reference in this particular setting?	What other influences does this frame of reference have in this particular setting?

Exercise 9.1.2. Fieldwork Sites and Frames of Reference

Fieldwork or clinical site:	Frame(s) of reference:
Types of clients (i.e., diagnoses or reason for referral):	How this frame of reference is applied with clients:
What would be common goals for intervention related to this frame of reference in this particular setting?	What other influences does this frame of reference have in this particular setting?

Exercise 9.1.3. Fieldwork Sites and Frames of Reference

Fieldwork or clinical site:	Frame(s) of reference:
Types of clients (i.e., diagnoses or reason for referral):	How this frame of reference is applied with clients:
What would be common goals for intervention related to this frame of reference in this particular setting?	What other influences does this frame of reference have in this particular setting?

Exercise 9.1.4. Fieldwork Sites and Frames of Reference

Fieldwork or clinical site:	Frame(s) of reference:
Types of clients (i.e., diagnoses or reason for referral):	How this frame of reference is applied with clients:
What would be common goals for intervention related to this frame of reference in this particular setting?	What other influences does this frame of reference have in this particular setting?

Summary

Occupational therapy clinical settings may be broadly characterized as traditional, nontraditional, or emerging and/or innovative, although this type of division is not always an effective description of a practice setting. The characteristics of these different types of settings can help you understand why some sites have greater flexibility than others, which is often based on what interventions can be provided in relation to reimbursement and funding sources. Discerning the differences and applying frames of reference to these settings may help you better understand your own work style preference and strengths. This understanding may also help you choose your first job after completing your fieldwork requirements.

Reference

Kramer, P., Blount, M.-L., & Blount, W. (2023). Occupation and occupational therapy. In M.-L. Blount & P. Kramer (with W. Blount) (Eds.), *The texture of life: Occupations and related activities* (5th ed., pp. 1–10). AOTA Press.

Chapter 10

Reimbursement, Documentation, and a Client-Centered Approach

TOPICS

- Understanding the business of coding and billing therapy services
- Recognizing that reimbursement pays your salary
- Knowing the importance of documentation
- Documenting with reimbursement in mind
- Making no assumptions
- Needing preauthorization
- Exploring who can do what
- Understanding that documentation equals proof of service
- Having the right code in the right place
- Making an error: What to do?
- Organizing using SOAP notes
- Ensuring well-written documentation

I had to review medical records whenever we received a subpoena for an outpatient occupational therapy medical record. The medical director or medical records department handled inpatient subpoenas. Usually, the subpoena related to what treatment was needed following an accident or injury and involved a client receiving compensation, insurance coverage, or damages from whoever was alleged to have caused the problem.

I hadn't realized it [receipt of subpoenas] occurred so often until I became an occupational therapy manager. I probably received four or five a month. I knew documentation was important for reimbursement, but it really hit home then just how many people would or might read what we had written in the medical records. From this experience, the therapy staff developed a new chart and documentation review that included EVERYONE who did documentation. Looking at random documentation to be sure we included all the points that insurance and legal reviewers were checking really improved everyone's documentation skills.

—BONNIE, occupational therapist (and co-author of this book) on my experience as an occupational therapy manager

Understanding the Business of Coding and Billing Therapy Services

Occupational therapy practitioners must prioritize providing high-quality client interventions, but receiving payment for services is also important. All practitioners, not just managers, must understand the business and legal aspects of health care. Successful practitioners are fiscally aware and understand the importance of a company's financial health. They understand that the business or facility as well as the paychecks for employees depend on several variables, including:

- costs of providing services
- appropriate documentation related to legal and ethical interventions
- current health care laws, legislation, and regulations
- requirements of third-party payers (e.g., insurance companies, Medicare, Medicaid).

Occupational therapy practitioners must consider their clients' needs and the financial realities of providing services. Costs must be covered, regulations followed, and requirements of payers met. The key elements are to be knowledgeable, aware, professional, and efficient. Efficiency is related to time, resources, and proof of effectiveness. An efficient practitioner does the following:

- works to achieve client goals in an optimal and appropriate amount of time
- develops a wide variety of intervention options (e.g., goes into treatment with flexibility and treatment options A, B, and C in case the client's needs differ from what was anticipated before treatment)
- delivers high-quality client education as well as interventions
- documents therapy accurately and concisely
- learns to use appropriate billing codes
- understands and adheres to payer requirements (just because you *can*, doesn't mean you *should*) and their relationship to your workplace guidelines
- keeps up-to-date on changes in coding requirements and other policies, procedures, and regulations that affect billing and reimbursement.

During your fieldwork, particularly in Level II, you will have opportunities to learn more about the business aspects of providing occupational therapy services to clients. Take advantage of these opportunities. Part of fieldwork is learning how your interventions are paid for and, therefore, how you will be paid.

Talk It Over With Your Fieldwork Supervisor

Talk with your fieldwork supervisor about the business of providing services. You might ask these questions:

- What techniques do occupational therapy practitioners use to be efficient without sacrificing the quality of therapy provided to their clients?
- What can I, as a student, do to contribute to appropriate billing and other business practices of the facility where I am doing my fieldwork?
- How do practitioners balance clients' needs and financial responsibilities, such as limited insurance coverage, rising service costs, and government regulations?
- How can I develop an understanding of the business of providing occupational therapy services?
- How do financial issues affect the daily work of occupational therapy practitioners?

Recognizing That Reimbursement Pays Your Salary

Most health care and other service fees are paid by someone other than the client. Known as *third-party payers,* these entities (mostly insurance companies or public programs) reimburse providers (e.g., individual therapists, companies, large facilities) for their services. Payments made by third-party payers to health care providers, including occupational therapy practitioners, depend on how well these health care professionals have documented their work based on an understanding of, and compliance with, payers' requirements and approved procedures.

Examples of major third-party payers include the following:

- **Traditional insurance.** Through health care policies, traditional insurance pays the fees for health care providers for individuals and/or bundled services; the client usually pays a copay. Examples of traditional insurers are Blue Cross/Blue Shield, Aetna, and other insurance companies that offer many variations in coverage, charge an assortment of premiums, differ widely in deductibles, pay for varied combinations of services, and pay providers. Health insurance is often offered with different levels of care: health maintenance organizations, preferred provider organizations, and point of service.
- **Medicare.** This is a federal insurance program that provides coverage for people ages 65 or older and those with certain disabilities. It is administered regionally by federally selected insurance companies called *fiscal intermediaries.* Fiscal

intermediaries may interpret Medicare slightly differently; this coverage can vary regionally. Not all older people are eligible for Medicare; eligibility is determined by a formula that is based on years of contribution to Medicare through employers.

- **Medicare Part A.** This part of Medicare covers hospitalization, home health care, skilled nursing care, and hospice care.
- **Medicare Part B.** This part covers outpatient services.
- **Medicare Part C, also known as Medicare Advantage.** This part combines Medicare Parts A and B and provides a minimum of the same coverage as do Parts A and B. Part C coverage is provided by private insurance companies funded and approved by Medicare.
- **Medicare Part D.** This part subsidizes some of the cost of Medicare-approved prescription medications for people already covered by Medicare programs.
- **Medigap policy.** This is supplemental insurance purchased by Medicare recipients to help pay the percentage of fees not covered by Medicare; it is often called coinsurance. Reimbursement varies widely among policies.
- **Medicaid.** This is a joint federal and state program that provides health and rehabilitative care for people who meet certain qualifications, such as low income and/or disability. Medicaid is a key funder of early intervention, school-based services, services for developmental disabilities, services for mental health, and other specialized services.
- **TRICARE** (formerly Civilian Health and Medical Program of the Uniformed Services [CHAMPUS]). TRICARE provides coverage for the dependents of active-duty military personnel, retired military personnel, and other groups associated with the military.
- **Workers' compensation insurance.** This is medical insurance coverage for employees who sustain work-related injuries, illness, or death. Compensation laws vary from state to state. Employers are assessed fees based on the number of employees, history of work-related injuries in the type of work, and records of a specific employer. Companies with more employees reporting injuries pay substantially higher premiums to the state fund from which workers' compensation claims are paid to injured workers.

Each of the aforementioned programs has different rules for what services will be authorized.

Many factors determine how and whether reimbursements are made. Never assume a client is covered by insurance. The following factors affect reimbursement:

- the setting in which services are provided, such as a hospital, long-term-care facility, outpatient clinic, community locations (e.g., school, community center), or the client's home
- the type of services provided by the occupational therapy practitioner (e.g., whether they meet the coverage criteria of the particular payer)
- details, such as specific approved dates for providing the services and use of proper terminology in the documentation

- the payer's understanding of occupational therapy, eligibility requirements, and procedures for requiring reimbursement, which vary widely with both agencies and insurance plans.

Insurance coverage for individuals and interpretation of that coverage by insurance companies are constantly changing. Medicare requirements also regularly change, especially when there are federal administration changes. Occupational therapy practitioners must stay up to date. It is highly recommended that you stay current by visiting the American Occupational Therapy Association (AOTA) website to review coding and billing resources (https://www.aota.org/practice/practice-essentials/coding). Table 10.1 offers some common terminology related to Medicare reimbursement.

TABLE 10.1. Medicare Reimbursement Language

Term	What It Is
CMS	This is a federal agency that oversees the Medicare and Medicaid programs.
CPT® codes (AMA, n.d.)	This reference book of numerical codes is used to identify and report medical procedures to be billed to insurance companies (except Medicare). It is published by the AMA (n.d.).
DMERCs	These private companies contract with Medicare to pay bills for durable medical equipment.
DRGs	This is a system that categorizes clients who have medically related diagnoses and treatment. Medicare pays a lump sum for inpatient stays based on DRGs rather than for an actual length of stay and individual services provided to a client.
Fee-for-service	This is a method of payment in which each specific service is reimbursed from a list of fees established for the health care provider.
Local coverage determination	These guidelines are set by Medicare contractors to help health care providers understand their implementation of Medicare coverage criteria and to submit acceptable claims for payment. These policies help identify acceptable descriptions of procedures and interventions provided by health care providers.

(Continued)

TABLE 10.1. Medicare Reimbursement Language *(Cont.)*

Term	What It Is
Medicare	This is nationwide health insurance for people ages 65 or older and certain people with disabilities or blindness. Part A covers inpatient hospital services, SNFs, medical equipment and supplies, and hospice care. Part B covers physicians, outpatient hospital services, medical equipment and supplies, and a variety of other services and supplies. Part C, also known as Medicare Advantage, is a combination of Parts A and B through some providers. Part D assists with covering prescription medications.
Medicare Advantage	Part C of Medicare, Medicare Advantage, consists of health plans run by Medicare-approved private insurance companies. Plans include Part A, Part B, and other coverage, such as prescription drugs.
Medicare contractors	These are organizations under contract to the government to process claims under Medicare, or organizations under contract with the state to process claims for Medicare.
NCCI	CMS (2025) publishes this quarterly manual with coding information for health care providers who work with Medicare and Medicaid clients. For example, the manual identifies therapeutic procedures that will not be reimbursed if performed for a client during the same session or the same day.
PDPM	This is a new case-mix classification model used under the SNF PPS for classifying SNF patients in a covered Part A stay.
PPS	This is a payment system in which the amounts paid are set regardless of what the provider charges (e.g., the SNF PPS pays a daily rate on the basis of the patient's condition).
RBRVS	This is a method the government uses to determine Medicare fee schedules. Each medical procedure is assigned a value that takes into account the time, skill, and overhead costs to provide the service or procedure.

Note. CMS = Centers for Medicare & Medicaid Services; *CPT*® = *Current Procedural Terminology*® codes; AMA = American Medical Association; DMERCs = durable medical equipment regional carriers; DRGs = diagnosis-related groups; SNFs = skilled nursing facilities; NCCI = National Correct Coding Initiative; PDPM = Patient-Driven Payment Model; SNF = skilled nursing facility; PPS = prospective payment system; RBRVS = Resource-Based Relative Value Scale.

Knowing the Importance of Documentation

Proper documentation serves a variety of purposes. As health care dollars become increasingly tight, documentation is a primary way to prove the value of occupational therapy intervention. Accurate documentation serves the following purposes:

- It provides an ongoing record for the occupational therapy practitioner.
- It is a way for the practitioner to share client information with other health care professionals involved in client interventions.
- It is a record of evidence-based practice.
- It helps ensure competence with regulatory agencies.
- It serves as a legal document that may be used to support continued occupational therapy services, prove the severity of client problems, and initiate necessary interventions related to malpractice suits or other litigation.
- It provides a source of information for facility accreditation reviews and visits.
- It improves cost control by eliminating the repetition of services.
- It provides information for quality improvement and utilization review.

Many people other than clinicians and members of the treatment team read the documentation. Third-party payers can review it, and payment for previously approved treatment sessions can be denied based on a review of documentation deemed insufficient or related to unauthorized procedures or activities done during therapy.

Clients also have the right to review their medical records. Medical and other records are frequently subpoenaed when questions related to care or treatment are provided. Keeping those potential readers in mind as you write documentation helps ensure that your notes are accurate and useful.

Documenting With Reimbursement in Mind

> Documentation of occupational therapy "is necessary whenever professional services are provided to a client."
>
> —AOTA (2018, p. 1)

Documentation is proof of services required for reimbursement. Three key elements help ensure that occupational therapy services will be reimbursed:

1. **Justification for the skilled services being delivered by an occupational therapy practitioner rather than an unskilled person.** The documentation must support that the intervention required knowledge and abilities specific to occupational therapy. This is especially important when Medicare is the payer. Sometimes, this is a matter of wording to prove the necessary knowledge level. Compare the meaning of the following two phrases: (a) "provided skilled instruction in donning shoes using assistive device"—this denotes teaching, which requires expertise; and

(b) "helped the client don shoes using assistive device"—this describes unskilled assistance that can be provided by an aide or family member.

2. **Documentation of functional outcome.** If a short-term goal and activity in a session focus on a performance component, such as improving balance, the purpose in terms of ultimate functional outcome ("shower safety") should be referenced and never assumed in the documentation.
3. **Documentation in terms of medical necessity.** Medicare and many managed care organizations approve only those services deemed medically necessary. Goals and treatment activities should be written in terms of payer-approved activities of daily living to support why they contribute to the approved intervention strategies.

Talk It Over With Your Fieldwork Supervisor

Talk with your fieldwork supervisor about the topic of documenting for reimbursement of occupational therapy services. Some questions to ask include:

- What is billable as occupational therapy in this facility?
- Some aspects of reimbursement vary regionally, by insurance company, and by diagnosis or purpose for referral to occupational therapy. Are there other factors to consider when documenting for reimbursement and continuing occupational therapy interventions?
- Are there words that I should avoid using in documentation at this agency?

Making No Assumptions

A good rule for dealing with payers, reimbursement requirements, and procedures is to not assume anything. The requirements can be complex and may be challenging to interpret. What might seem appropriate services for the client may not be in the client's specific policy. Some payers may need explanations about occupational therapy in language the insurers understand.

Remember: This is an opportunity to educate payers, not a time to get angry or defensive because they are not familiar with your profession! Reimbursement can be denied because a procedure is inappropriately coded in a computerized billing system, which is a clerical error. An insurance company may deny certain codes for occupational therapy, or the provider may need more information. AOTA (2025) is continually working to educate the government and insurance companies about the nature of occupational therapy to ensure proper reimbursement. This work is what part of our professional association dues support and is an essential reason to maintain membership throughout your career.

Never assume that what seems right or makes sense for a client will be approved or reimbursed. Consider this example: A client who sustained a cerebral vascular accident returned home after a month of institutional care and is using a wheelchair and is unable to drive. Relatives transported the client to outpatient therapy at a hospital for continued services. When the client requested a home visit from an occupational therapist to help them set up their kitchen and teach them to safely cook using adaptive equipment and techniques, the insurance company denied coverage for in-home intervention. The insurance company reasoned that in-home visits were unnecessary if the client could get to the hospital. The occupational therapy practitioner had to provide additional documentation explaining that the in-home assessment and training for equipment would increase the client's independence and safety.

Sometimes part, but not all, of a service is reimbursable. This can be confusing for both the client and occupational therapy practitioner. Sometimes, the insurance company interprets coverage such that when any part of a client's treatment is denied, all treatment payments are denied. Some insurance plans will not reimburse for assistive devices yet will pay for the therapy to train clients to use the devices and for some materials needed to provide the training. Medicare will not reimburse some procedures if performed during the same treatment session as other procedures; these are known as *mutually exclusive procedures,* and the exact procedures vary. Practitioners need to stay current with coding standards, and it is best to consult the National Correct Coding Initiative (NCCI; see Table 10.1), published quarterly by the Centers for Medicare & Medicaid Services (2025).

Another source of confusion is that some insurance companies have policies with similar names. For example, Blue Cross/Blue Shield provides a variety of plans and options to employers and subscribers, but the policies could be confused because of the names (e.g., Blue Advantage vs. Blue Care). Therefore, clients with the same insurance company may have very different coverage depending on their particular policy.

Level II fieldwork students need to know the reimbursement requirements that affect their clients. Never imply to clients that their insurance company will cover specific treatments, equipment, devices, or other services. Sometimes, in an effort to be helpful, health care personnel encourage clients to not worry about financial aspects but, rather, to focus on getting better. Helping the client or responsible family member obtain information about their coverage can decrease anxiety and increase the client's ability to use available services. "Don't worry" comments can be a disservice to clients who may later learn they are financially responsible for services they cannot afford. Know the designated professional in your setting with whom the client can discuss insurance and reimbursement issues. Even experienced clinicians can't know it all.

Talk It Over With Your Fieldwork Supervisor

Talk with your fieldwork supervisor about reimbursement issues. You might ask these questions:

- Do you [fieldwork supervisor] have examples of common reimbursement pitfalls about which I should be aware?
- What are your recommendations for learning about payers and reimbursement policies and procedures?
- Does the agency or department have written resources to help me learn more about reimbursement issues related to this specific site or client population?

Needing Preauthorization

Rehabilitation services usually must be approved before working with a client, a practice known as *preauthorization*. Without preauthorization, reimbursement may be, and often is, denied, even for treatment that might have received preauthorization. Preauthorization is typically given for a specific number of sessions, specific time periods, and specific types of treatment. The clinician needs to be fully informed about preauthorization to stay within the approved number, dates approved, or types of services that have been approved.

Preauthorization may be approved in clusters of services. For example, say a client is initially approved to receive three sessions per week for 6 weeks. The occupational therapy practitioner determines that additional sessions are needed to achieve the client's goals, so another preauthorization is required. The practitioner would then submit a request for additional sessions toward the end of the 6-week authorized services. Starting the necessary paperwork early in the treatment period can avoid or eliminate a gap in services while waiting for another authorization. However, requesting additional sessions too soon may cause a denial because treatment time is still available to make significant changes related to the client's needs. It's all about timing and good communication.

Most clients do not fully understand their insurance coverage until they need it. Many agencies have specialized personnel who check client insurance coverage and help insurance companies understand the purpose of the referral. Sometimes, the occupational therapy practitioner is responsible for ensuring that the services being provided will be covered. An important part of delivering good client service is being informed about specific agency procedures. Become familiar with your agency's policies!

Exploring Who Can Do What

Documentation of treatment and procedures performed by fieldwork students must be cosigned by the supervisor, who is legally responsible for the student's work. You, the student, are operating under your supervisor's license! Students must sign the documentation for their services, which a supervisor must then cosign. Ask your agency or supervisor for specific procedures because of slight variations among agencies.

Occupational therapy assistants cannot initiate treatment but may contribute to initial evaluations, which the occupational therapist interprets. Treatment planning, changes in treatment plan, reevaluation, and discharge planning and notes must be signed by the occupational therapist supervising the occupational therapy assistant. Based on Medicare interpretation, occupational therapy assistants are granted more freedom related to treatment decisions and supervision than other assistants, such as nursing and physical therapy. Occupational therapy practitioners must be familiar with these differences and where they are stated in Medicare regulations. It is your responsibility to be informed of Medicare and state regulations!

The forms and formats used to document occupational therapy services vary widely from facility to facility and state to state. Knowing some of the common requirements for all settings is helpful for documentation. Keep the following rules in mind:

- Include all required information.
- Be concise! (If you use the adjective *very*, you aren't being concise! Quantify it.)
- Be sure the client's name and identifying numbers appear on every page.
- Always record information on the client's chart after providing services—never before. Write documentation as soon as possible after the event to maintain accuracy. When a time delay occurs, make notes to yourself related to everything that needs to be documented.
- If writing rather than typing into a chart, write legibly. Remember: This is a legal document.
- Spell correctly, being especially careful with easily confused words, such as *dysphasia* and *dysphagia*. If necessary, carry a sheet on your clipboard or in a pocket with the correct spelling of words that give you problems—and watch out for computer spell-check corrections that change your meaning!
- Use abbreviations only when doing so is acceptable to your facility. Most facilities have a list of acceptable abbreviations. Take time to review that list and keep it handy when writing documentation. When in doubt, write it out!
- Use only acceptable and professional terminology.
- If providing handwritten notes, use only black pens—never colored ink or a pencil. If you have written a note in error, draw a single line through the text, correct the error, and add your initials. Never strike out multiple lines and never use correction fluid or tape.
- Record the time and date of entries. Computerized documentation will usually do this for you.
- As a student, be sure your supervisor approves your drafted documentation *before* writing in a client's chart.

Understanding That Documentation Equals Proof of Service

Written documentation proves the services were provided and justifies the need for each service. Providers demand accountability, and documentation is the primary and legal way to demonstrate that need and accountability. Improper documentation, even if it is the result of ignorance, can be grounds for denial of service and denial of payment for services already provided. Deliberate misrepresentation in documentation is unethical, according to the AOTA (2020a) *Code of Ethics*, and may be considered fraud or grounds for losing licensure. The National Health Care Anti-Fraud Association (2024) "estimates that the financial losses due to health care fraud are in the tens of billions of dollars each year" (para. 2).

The forms you will use for documentation will vary widely among facilities, agencies, insurance companies, and Medicare intermediaries. You must document similar treatment to meet the payers' requirements in different formats. Completeness and accuracy are essential to all who review or use the medical records of treatment. Your fieldwork supervisors will be well versed in their facility's needs.

Having the Right Code in the Right Place

Being familiar with procedural terminology codes and acceptable diagnoses for occupational therapy intervention helps to create acceptable and reimbursable services. *Procedure coding* is the use of a predetermined numerical system for identifying diagnoses and treatments; it also identifies reimbursement rates for the service provided. The primary source for procedural codes is a manual published by the American Medical Association (n.d.) and updated annually: the *Current Procedural Terminology®* (*CPT®*). Agencies using this coding system will have copies of the *CPT* book in their billing offices. Many third-party payers use the *CPT* codes even if their reimbursement differs from Medicare.

If you work with Medicare or Medicaid clients, another source of information is the aforementioned NCCI. This quarterly manual (CMS, 2025) identifies coding errors that negatively affect Medicare reimbursement and compliance. The NCCI is the source for the mutually exclusive procedures mentioned earlier in this chapter. It also includes comprehensive and component procedures, which are combinations of codes that will not be reimbursed when performed on the same date for a client. Specific amounts paid by Medicare vary from state to state and region to region. Correctly coding a diagnosis, reason for referral, or procedure (i.e., specific intervention) can make the difference between being reimbursed and being denied. The documentation for your interventions must support the codes assigned. Coding has been called an art that is mastered through both study and experience.

Talk It Over With Your Fieldwork Supervisor

Talk with your fieldwork supervisor about procedure coding by asking questions like these:

- Which codes are most commonly used in this facility? Why are those the most commonly used codes?
- What recommendations can you [fieldwork supervisor] give me about coding accurately?

Making an Error: What to Do?

If you make an error when charting (this happens to everyone at one time or another), check first with your supervisor for directions related to that specific facility on how to handle the error. Most electronic health records have mechanisms built into the system to automatically strike through and correct documentation for you per facility guidelines. If using paper charts, do *not* erase, do not use correction tape or fluid, and do not just mark over the incorrect entry; these types of corrections on a legal document are considered illegal record alterations. The general rules for correcting mistakes are, as mentioned earlier in the "Exploring Who Can Do What Section," to draw a single line through the incorrect portion, write "error" (or the facility-designated word or abbreviation), write the correct information as near to the original entry as possible, and include the date of the correction and your initials. If you write an entry in the wrong client's chart, draw a line through the entry, write "wrong chart," add your initials, and date the correction.

Talk It Over With Your Fieldwork Supervisor

Talk with your fieldwork supervisor about documenting effectively by asking questions like these:

- What advice do you [fieldwork supervisor] have regarding effective documentation?
- Have you developed strategies for writing accurate documentation in a timely manner?
- How can I become more concise and succinct with documentation?

Organizing Using SOAP Notes

Documentation can be organized into various formats. The SOAP notes format—subjective, objective, assessment, plan—is a technique that can help you organize client information and separate it into these four important categories (Sames, 2015). Given the many variations in documentation because of differences in requirements for schools, hospitals, nebula health settings, and community- or home-based interventions, you may not end up using the SOAP notes technique. However, you can apply the logical division of content illustrated by that technique by documenting your interventions with clients into those general four categories.

Subjective Information

Subjective information is qualitative and may refer to the client's conversation about problems, complaints, life circumstances, goals, current performance, limitations, or other issues (Sames, 2015). Subjective information is relevant to therapy. It is a way to reference information or comments that may be helpful but cannot be verified or measured by the health care practitioner. Subjective information in an occupational therapy setting may include statements given by the client, family member, or other significant person (e.g., caregiver) that convey information about or reflect on

- previous or current function;
- pain and physical limitations;
- mental functioning;
- living arrangements;
- interests and lifestyle preferences;
- strengths, such as the client's abilities or support system; and
- goals and desired outcomes of therapy.

Client behaviors, such as missing appointments or refusing to cooperate during therapy, might also be noted in the subjective section of documentation. In this section, you may summarize information provided by the client or quote the client directly (e.g., "The client stated, '[client quote].'"). When recording subjective information supplied by the client, family, or friends, quote them as exactly as possible. Do not try interpreting what you *think* they might mean.

The following are examples of what might be included as subjective information:

- The client stated, "I feel tingling in my fingers."
- The client's husband stated, "Marcia seems to have lost interest in doing her exercises, and that isn't like her."

Novice occupational therapy practitioners often feel they must talk with the client until they obtain something relevant for subjective comments. Sames (2015) has reminded health care practitioners that if nothing is relevant to report, then nothing needs to be documented. If the facility or occupational therapy fieldwork educator expects something in each category, then you can place a circle with a line through it in this section to show that subjective information has been addressed and that you have nothing to report.

Social content should not be documented in this section. Instead, use open-ended questions to obtain relevant information from clients about their history, problems, interests, values related to outcomes, support system, living situation, and goals for therapy. Questions that help focus the conversation on treatment needs include: "What do you want to be able to do?" "What stops you from doing that?" "Who helps you at home?"

A common mistake health care practitioners make is writing down something clients say about themselves rather than consolidating the information and extracting the relevant content. If several statements refer to the same problem, concisely summarize, rather than list, each one.

Objective Information

Objective information is quantifiable and includes treatment results (the results themselves, *not* an interpretation of the results), measurements, and the occupational therapy practitioner's observations. You record objective observations; that is, what you saw—akin to a recording—rather than what you may have inferred or interpreted. For example, writing "Client is upset" is subjective, whereas "Client was crying and refused to participate in therapy" is objective. The emphasis is on how the client performs during therapy, not on the activities in which the client participates. Avoid dwelling on negatives; instead, report strengths or weaknesses in performance.

Objective information may include

- demographics;
- past medical history relevant to goals;
- referral information, such as physician's orders;
- performance related to the specific problem for which the referral has been made;
- standardized or criteria-referenced test results; and
- reports based on the occupational therapy practitioner's direct observations (not their interpretations).

Assessment

Assessment refers to the occupational therapist's interpretation, conclusions, or opinions based on the content in the subjective and objective sections. It is the meaning suggested by the data gathered and documented. An *interpretation* is not the same as a *diagnosis,* which is the medical description of the cause and symptoms of a condition. Information from the subjective and objective sections is analyzed in the assessment section (Sames, 2015).

The assessment section may include

- the client's tolerance of intervention techniques,
- a summary of achieved goals determined and supported by the objective data,
- the potential of the client to meet current or future goals, and
- areas of the *Occupational Therapy Practice Framework* (*Framework* AOTA, 2020b) on which intervention may be focused.

New information about the client should not be included in the assessment section but should go in either the subjective or objective sections—whichever is appropriate and relevant.

Plan

Plan refers to the client record documenting the type of intervention selected to achieve the client's targeted outcomes. The plan section might include the following information:

- recommended intervention strategies
- long-term goals related to the functional areas in the *Framework* (AOTA, 2020b)
- short-term goals specifically related to achieving each long-term goal
- time frames: how long or how many treatment sessions are anticipated
- frequency of treatment: how often the client will be seen (e.g., daily, 2 times per week)
- who will provide the treatment.

Talk It Over With Your Fieldwork Supervisor

Goals should always be supported by content included in the subjective and objective sections of the client's record and interpreted in the assessment. All of these content areas should come together to support the goals.

Ask your supervisor these questions:

- Are particular phrases often used in the facility to introduce goals, such as: "The client would benefit from [intervention]," or "[intervention] may help move the client to a lesser level of care"?
- Do you [fieldwork supervisor] recommend using those types of phrases?
- What is the common practice in this agency?

Ensuring Well-Written Documentation

You can be great at client interaction and providing successful interventions and treatment, but without accurate, well-written, and appropriate documentation, you and your agency will not get reimbursement for your services. Skill in documentation is essential to you and your agency. See Exhibit 10.1 for fundamental elements required for good documentation. Next, complete Exercise 10.1 to better understand well-written documentation

EXHIBIT 10.1. Fundamental Elements of Documentation

- Client's full name and case number on each page of documentation
- Date and type of occupational therapy contact
- Identification of type of documentation, agency, and department name
- Occupational therapy signature with first name or initial, last name, and professional designation
- When applicable on notes or reports, signature of the recorder directly at the end of the note without space left between the body of the note and the signature
- Countersignature by an occupational therapist on documentation written by students or occupational therapy assistants when required by law or by the facility
- Acceptable terminology defined within the boundaries of the setting

- Abbreviation usage as acceptable within the boundaries of the setting
- When no facility requirements are listed, errors are corrected by drawing a single line through an error and initialing the correction; correction fluid or tape and erasures are not acceptable
- Adherence to professional standards of terminology used to document occupational therapy
- Disposal of records within law and agency requirements
- Compliance with confidentiality standards
- Compliance with legal and agency requirements of storage of records

---

Exercise 10.1. Learning by Example: Well-Written Documentation

Ask your supervisor to provide examples of well-written documentation specific to the site where you are doing your fieldwork. Then analyze the way that content is presented. What you'll be doing here is similar to completing chart reviews, as is done in every health care facility.

• What makes the documentation easy to read and understand?
• How does the writer include important information without being too wordy?
• What type of information is included in each section of the documentation?

Suggested documentation content specific to occupational therapy is as follows, in five parts:

1. **Evaluation**
   - client information
   - referral information
   - occupational profile
   - assessments used and results
   - analysis of occupational performance
   - summary and analysis
   - recommendations

2. **Reevaluation report** (the frequency of reevaluation depends on the needs of the setting and the client's progress)
    - client information
    - occupational profile
    - reevaluation results
    - summary and analysis
    - recommendations
3. **Intervention**
    - client information
    - intervention goals
    - intervention approaches and types of interventions to be used
    - services delivery mechanisms
    - plan for discharge
    - outcome measures
    - name of professionals responsible and date of the plan
4. **Progress report**
    - client information
    - summary of services provided
    - current client performance
    - plan or recommendations
5. **Outcome or discharge**
    - client information
    - summary of intervention process
    - recommendations (AOTA, 2020b)

In some facilities, the initial evaluation and discharge reports are included in one document to help reviewers easily compare the effectiveness of interventions. Other occupational therapy practitioners and reviewers may use the report.

Talk It Over With Your Fieldwork Supervisor

Ask your supervisor for detailed information about the specific documentation requirements for your fieldwork setting. Request and be open to feedback on your documentation. Remember that this feedback is not just about you but focuses on enabling the best interventions and reimbursement for the client to achieve occupational goals. If service is provided and denied, the client becomes responsible for out-of-pocket payment for therapy!

Summary

Reimbursement from third-party payers, whether private or government agencies, is the most common form of reimbursement for most health care services. Further, the number and variety of requirements change. Maintaining reimbursement for occupational therapy services requires both attention to documentation and support of AOTA, which is attentive to and stays up-to-date with legislative issues that can affect occupational therapy reimbursement.

Accurate and complete documentation benefits your clients by contributing to quality occupational therapy. It benefits your employer by supporting your agency, and it benefits you by providing your salary. The occupational therapy practitioner must know the specific requirements for reimbursement, and the practitioner is responsible for educating the third-party payer. The third-party payer won't reimburse for services they either don't understand or don't value. It is our individual and professional responsibility not to get frustrated when people don't understand occupational therapy. See those moments as an opportunity to educate third-party payers, family, and even coworkers in other disciplines about the purpose and value of occupational therapy.

References

American Medical Association. (n.d.). *CPT® (Current Procedural Terminology).* https://www.ama-assn.org/amaone/cpt-current-procedural-terminology

American Occupational Therapy Association. (2018). Guidelines for documentation of occupational therapy. *American Journal of Occupational Therapy, 72*(Suppl. 2), 7212410010. https://doi.org/10.5014/ajot.2018.72S203

American Occupational Therapy Association. (2020a). AOTA 2020 occupational therapy code of ethics. *American Journal of Occupational Therapy, 74*(Suppl. 3), 7413410005. https://doi.org/10.5014/ajot.2020.74S3006

American Occupational Therapy Association. (2020b). Occupational therapy practice framework: Domain and process (4th ed.). *American Journal of Occupational Therapy, 74*(Suppl. 2), 7412410010. https://doi.org/10.5014/ajot.2020.74S2001

American Occupational Therapy Association. (2025). *Advocacy issues in focus.* https://www.aota.org/advocacy/issues

Centers for Medicare & Medicaid Services. (2025). *Medicare NCCI policy manual.* https://www.cms.gov/files/document/2025nccimedicarepolicymanualcompletepdf.pdf

National Health Care Anti-Fraud Association. (2024). *The challenge of health care fraud.* https://www.nhcaa.org/tools-insights/about-health-care-fraud/the-challenge-of-health-care-fraud/

Sames, K. M. (2015). *Documenting occupational therapy practice* (3rd ed.). Pearson.

Chapter 11

Making Clients Your Priority: Transitioning From School Assignments to Therapeutic Relationships and Interventions

TOPICS

- Shifting perspectives
- Developing therapeutic relationships: Respect for clients
- Understanding communication variations: Client, professional, and casual
- Working with challenging clients
- Taking care of yourself

I knew there probably was a problem when I covered some patients for a new [occupational] therapist. The patient seemed to know all about the personal life of the therapist for whom I was covering. I figured it meant that she'd done all the talking when it seemed like there should have been more information and assessment of the patient. I wasn't sure what to do, but I focused on the patient and completing the assessment. Then I went to my supervisor because I knew I could ask her if I should say something. She helped me deal with how I felt and then said it was something she would handle. I really believed there were some things that the patient knew that had no business being shared, especially during the patient's time. It didn't seem like a very professional relationship had been established. The supervisor reassured me that I understood patient-focused treatment and had recognized a potential problem.

—JENNIFER, new occupational therapy assistant

Shifting Perspectives

Academic settings focus on your individual performance. Your progress as a student is measured by test scores, the quality of your papers and projects, and the demonstration of skills. When you become an occupational therapy practitioner, however, your success is measured in terms of the performance of others: your clients. Are clients achieving the goals set with them? The focus has shifted from you to them. By continually asking yourself, "Are the client's needs being met as I work with them to achieve their targeted outcomes?" thinking in terms of client performance will become second nature.

Developing Therapeutic Relationships: Respect for Clients

The therapeutic relationship begins with the occupational therapy practitioner's natural desire to work with clients and to shift their perspective from self-achievement to client achievement. This shift in perspective is complemented by many other elements as Figure 11.1 illustrates.

An important characteristic of the entry-level practitioner is the ability to consider all the variables shown in Figure 11.1 when engaging in the therapeutic relationship. Level I and Level II fieldwork provide opportunities to work with a variety of clients and to observe and begin to understand how these factors influence your work with your clients. A good starting point is to compare your beliefs about wellness with those of others; Exercise 11.1 can help you do that. Then do Exercise 11.2, which helps you explore what variables may influence your work with specific clients.

With its focus on function and increasing the ability to maximize one's independence and quality of life, occupational therapy embodies the notion of working *with* and not *for* the client. Occupational therapy, by its very nature, is collaborative. You may, however, find yourself confronted by clients who want and expect you to assist them more than is beneficial for their learning and achievement of therapeutic goals. Clients may have been over-helped in an acute setting, such as when the nursing staff provides care to many clients or by well-meaning parents of pediatric clients, because it is much faster to do things for clients than to encourage them to do things for themselves. In occupational therapy interventions, though, the client should be encouraged to do things for themselves. The occupational therapy practitioner's goal is to promote independent function. It takes longer to encourage someone to do something themself, but doing so teaches independence instead of helplessness.

Some cultures expect assistance to be provided to those who are sick or to people with disabilities; to withhold assistance is a sign of disrespect. What one person considers enabling behavior that fosters unhealthy dependency, someone else may consider to be appropriate, loving care. Helping clients and their families understand the purposes and advantages of therapy is part of establishing a therapeutic relationship—and may help you recognize and appreciate how others view what is important in life. Goals are useful only if clients and their families and support networks understand them and if the goals meet the clients' needs.

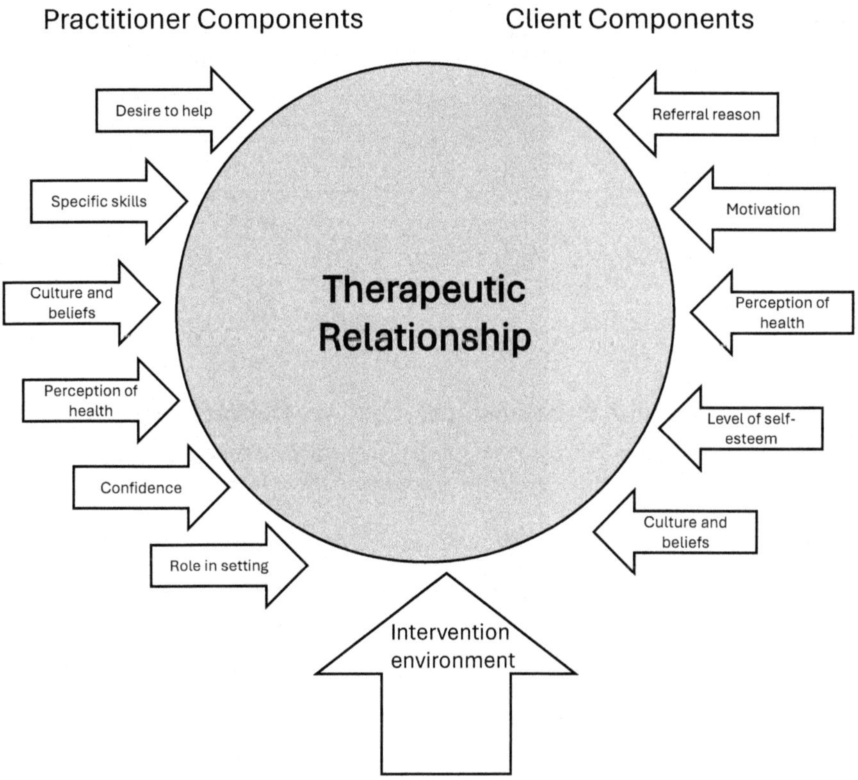

FIGURE 11.1. Culturally responsive care.

Exercise 11.1. Whose Views?

Note. Before beginning this exercise, consult with your fieldwork supervisor, who is responsible for your interactions with clients, and secure their approval.

Choose **two** clients whose views about health might be different from your own. Ask appropriate nonjudgmental questions, listen actively, and observe carefully.

The following are examples of appropriate questions:

- What do you do to help you stay healthy?
- What do you usually do when you are not feeling well?
- To whom do you go first when seeking help with health problems?
- What do you think are the main causes of health problems?

Compare the views of the clients with yours. How might the differences, if any, influence your work as an occupational therapy practitioner?

Things the two clients have said:	Comparisons with your own beliefs:

Things the two clients have said:	Comparisons with your own beliefs:

Exercise 11.2. Therapeutic Relationships: What Are the Variables?

Note. Before beginning this exercise, consult with your fieldwork supervisor, who is responsible for your interactions with clients, and secure their approval.

Choose **two** clients and fill in as many of the variables from Figure 11.1 as possible that you believe might influence the formation of therapeutic relationships with these two clients.

Client 1:	**Variables:**
Client 2:	**Variables:**

Understanding Communication Variations: Client, Professional, and Casual

Genuine concern for the client's well-being is the touchstone of respect. It is an important part of any valued relationship; however, with clients, it is a vital part of healing. A friendship may shift back and forth in concerns for each other, but the clinician–client relationship tips toward focusing on the client. Concern begins with *empathy,* a striving to understand the client's experience from the client's point of view. Disability, disease, and injury almost always result in some loss: loss of independence and loss of one's usual role in society, status, home life, comfort, expectation of physical pain, comfort, and privacy.

Reactions can vary as widely as the losses for the individual affected and their loved ones (see Exercise 11.3). Some clients experience high levels of stress, loss of self-esteem or identity, anger, frustration, and depression, any of which can prevent improvement or acceptance of new permanent or temporary limitations. These reactions, combined with the uniqueness of each client, can challenge the skills and enrich the experiences of the new occupational therapy practitioner. Strive to work effectively with each client, honoring their autonomy, so they can return to a lifestyle they value, even when you may not agree with their choices. Part of your role is to offer alternative ways to a lifestyle that the client values. Knowing how to respond to

Exercise 11.3. Thinking About Loss

Note. Before beginning this exercise, consult with your fieldwork supervisor, who is responsible for your interactions with clients, and secure their approval.

Think about the types of loss experienced by **two** of your clients. Consider where they are in their rehabilitation process:

- Have they learned new coping skills?
- Are their old coping skills helping or hindering their progress?
- How might you handle the experience of loss?
- What do you think your reactions might be?

Clients	Consider what your own feelings might be if you were in the client's situation:
Client 1	
Client 2	

every client you encounter is unrealistic and is why constant learning is essential to success as a clinician—even for experienced clinicians (see Exercise 11.4 to explore clients' challenges and needs).

Enhancing the quality of time spent with the client can express respect and concern (see Exercises 11.5 and 11.6). Chapter 4 discussed ways in which occupational therapy practitioners can maximize their time with clients with a focus on increasing efficiency. The reminders in the list that follows are similar, but they are offered in the context of compassion and personal attention. They are nonverbal ways to say, "You are worthy of my time" and "You have my attention":

- Approach the client slowly and professionally, even if you hurried to the area.
- Seek a quiet place and remove as many distractions as possible, including things you bring into the environment—not just what is already there.
- Introduce and explain yourself: The client may have forgotten you, which discipline you represent, or what you may expect from them.
- Never mention how busy you are; the client should be the center of your attention for this time.
- Make eye contact with the client and use eye contact in culturally responsive ways.
- Do your best to protect the time you have from interruptions. Put your beeper or cell phone on vibration mode and take care of personal business before or after your client-focused time. Remember: The client is paying for your time and attention!

Exercise 11.4. Each Client Is Unique

Note. Before beginning this exercise, consult with your fieldwork supervisor, who is responsible for your interactions with clients, and secure their approval.

Describe what appear to be the needs and challenges of **two** of your clients. If you were in their place, consider these questions:

- How might you respond to these needs and challenges?
- What would you hope to receive from occupational therapy interventions?
- Do you think these clients have the same expectations you would have?

Clients	Consider what your own feelings might be if you were in the client's situation:
Client 1	
Client 2	

Exercise 11.5. Reflection on Focusing on Clients

Reflect on your actions with clients:

- Are you able to attend fully to the client during interactions?
- What techniques have you developed or discovered to help you focus attention on your clients?

Problems you have had or observed	Possible solutions

Exercise 11.6. Reflecting on Interactions With Clients

Think about recent interactions with your clients. Consider the following:

- Do you believe you were able to establish rapport?
- How were you able to enhance their feelings of self-worth? What worked for you? How might you have done better?
- What might you try next time in working with these or other clients?

What problems occurred?	What worked or could have improved the interactions?

Health care communication is special. It is one-sided with the clinician focused on the client. Health care communication includes interactions between health care providers and between providers and the client. Unlike casual conversation, the therapeutic exchange of information is the basis of this type of communication: It is purposeful, usually time limited, and client focused. Taylor (2020) described therapeutic communication as involving both verbal and nonverbal cues (e.g., body language, facial expression), active listening (see Chapter 6), and seeking and responding to feedback to give clients a sense of structure and direction. Although Taylor's model focuses on provider–client communication, the same elements are key to good communication with other health care providers and team members and assessing the accuracy of information provided through documentation.

Sames (2015) cautioned about the choice of potentially loaded words or irrelevant content, particularly in documentation, and provided this example: The phrases "denies symptoms" or "refuses treatment" sound judgmental and biased. Use the subjective portion of the note to share what the client actually said and avoid making interpretations about the client's experience. Become aware of words that are loaded with negative or unintended meanings. Documentation should provide quantifiable information, not judgment!

Working With Challenging Clients

According to Haddad et al. (2023), health professionals have definite ideas about what constitutes a "good" client: Good clients want to get better, make an effort to get better, and appreciate the help they receive in their efforts to get better. They respect health professionals and follow all the recommendations prescribed for their care. In reality, health care providers' perceptions of a "good" client can be detrimental to client care. Research shows that this disparity between a provider's perceptions of a "good client" and patients' actual experiences and perspectives is a major problem in health care (Creel & Yinger, 2002). Health care providers may prioritize efficiency, financial stability, and adherence to protocols over what clients may value, such as compassionate care, personalized attention, and feeling understood. This discrepancy can lead to misunderstandings, miscommunication, and poor patient outcomes (Akhavan & Tillgren, 2015; Ferreira et al., 2023). If clients repeatedly experience this in their health care interactions, it's no wonder that they may be apprehensive about or resist the therapeutic or rehabilitative process.

Even knowing that these disparities between health care providers and clients exist, it can still be frustrating for occupational therapy practitioners who have spent years studying and preparing to help others maximize their function or improve their quality of life to be thwarted by the clients themselves when providing interventions aimed at helping them improve. Clients may seem uncooperative for many reasons, including fear, anger, frustration, pain, confusion, distrust, and depression as a result of their condition and limitations. In a few cases, being a client means receiving attention that they may find uncomfortable. Review the exercises in this chapter and try to understand your clients' perspectives. Two questions to remember when working with clients are: What underlies this behavior? and What can I do to encourage more constructive behavior?

As a new occupational therapy practitioner, you are likely to have high hopes and will make strong efforts to help every one of your clients. Exercise 11.7 can prepare you to work with difficult clients.

Exercise 11.7. What Is Difficult? The Truth of the Matter

At some point, you will encounter clients who challenge you. It's natural to have a variety of feelings in reaction to such clients, including doubt, frustration, annoyance, and even anger.

As you complete this exercise, consider what it might look like for a client to express each of the problems listed and think about what your reactions—both spontaneous and therapeutic—might be. It may be helpful to explore the feelings you have experienced or may experience in the future.

Consider how you might feel about, and work with, clients who:	What are your reactions—both spontaneous and therapeutic?
Don't want to help themselves	
Complain about everything	
Are very demanding or want everything done for them	
Don't practice good cleanliness and good personal hygiene	
Don't show respect to others	

Refuse to take responsibility for themselves but blame others, the circumstances, and so on for their condition	
Have socially unacceptable conditions, such as drug addiction	
Want you to assume the role of "good friend" rather than helping professional.	

Clients are not friends or relatives. You build professional therapeutic relationships to help your clients maximize their skills to succeed in their own lives. Before you encounter a client whom you perceive as difficult or frustrating, it is helpful to plan your responses using the proactive technique in Exercise 11.8. Having answers at the ready is essential in difficult situations when time limitations require immediate responses and professional behavior and may include safety issues for both you and the client. Like goals, having this list can make it easier to deal with challenging interactions.

The answers to the questions in Exercise 11.8 may change with experience. Your professional response must mediate your personal response. Sometimes client responses inadvertently hit personal trigger points. Part of professional growth and behavior is to maintain professional responses and client-focused behavior. Consider the following situation-based questions and then see how the tips for dealing with tough client comments in Exhibit 11.1 might pertain:

- Do you find yourself reacting emotionally to certain types of clients? In what ways? How would you describe those ways?
- What might be the cause of your reaction: something in your background or an experience? Or does the client remind you of someone?
- Is it easy for you to recognize your emotional reactions? Or do you need help from trusted peers if you feel you may be emotionally reacting to a client in a negative way?
- How can you recognize your limitations? What can you do about them so they don't negatively affect client interactions?

Exercise 11.8. Reasons for Dealing With Challenging Situations

Answer these questions so you can review, revise, and reflect on them when you encounter a difficult client.

Question	My answers
What were my reasons for becoming an occupational therapy practitioner?	
How do these reasons influence my relationships with clients?	
How have I *effectively* stepped back and temporarily removed myself from difficult situations in positive ways, and will these work in a *professional* situation?	

EXHIBIT 11.1. Quick Tips for Working With Challenging Clients

- Focus on the client's behavior.
- Look for underlying reasons for the behavior.
- Look for ways to engage the client in making decisions, as appropriate, about their treatment. Don't make the decision open ended; instead, provide specific choices.
- Have realistic expectations of yourself and recognize your own limitations.
- Be aware of your emotional responses to clients.
- Keep in mind that one of the best things you can offer your clients is a professional perspective, not an emotional one.

Talk It Over With Your Fieldwork Supervisor

Discuss the topic of demanding clients with your supervisor and ask them these questions:

- What experiences have you had with clients who have challenged you?
- Are there cases or situations for which I can prepare?
- What advice can you [fieldwork supervisor] offer about separating personal feelings from professional responsibilities?
- Do you have techniques that you have found helpful in working with particular types of clients?

If you are currently working with clients whom you consider to be difficult, discuss your interactions with your supervisors and ask them for feedback and suggestions.

Keep in mind:

- A therapeutic relationship is not a friendship. Be aware that strong feelings—both positive and negative—can occur from time to time. Learn to recognize and deal with those feelings in a professional manner.
- A therapeutic relationship is time limited and is directed by specific goals. Stay focused on the goals so that you can concentrate on the interventions that are in the client's best interest.
- A therapeutic relationship is always client focused. It is not about you; you are the coach or catalyst for the client's success.
- Remember that genuine caring is best expressed through applying your professional skills to help clients achieve their goals.

Sometimes, you will need to negotiate. No one is always right, and the best solutions are often a combination of several ideas. The art of negotiation is the ability to create win–win solutions. If your client does not want to do something, listen carefully and communicate. You may have a significant reason for your approach and can give a simple explanation that may change how they feel. Conversely, the client's resistance might be well-grounded and related to pain or lack of meaning. You can only find this out if you listen! Negotiation involves compromise. It isn't about power or control; it's about results and achieving health and quality-of-life goals for your clients.

Taking Care of Yourself

Making clients your priority includes taking care of yourself. If you don't, you may lack the energy and focus to provide high-quality occupational therapy, which can negatively affect your close relationships with family and friends. Proper self-care can increase your effectiveness in providing good client care. Respect for others begins with regard for the self. Level II fieldwork can be demanding of your time and energy, so taking care of yourself with proper nutrition, adequate exercise, and stress relief techniques will ultimately pay off for both you and your clients.

Haddad et al. (2023) described the clinical portion of education for health care providers as experiencing new smells, sounds, and sights combined with new tasks to present a weighty challenge to the best of classroom students. Taking time for solitude and reflection may help you process and evaluate the meaning of new experiences and reenergize yourself physically and mentally. Time invested in replenishing the spirit will benefit both you and others and increase the value produced and received in Level II fieldwork experiences.

An important part of taking care of yourself is understanding and accepting the realities, along with the joys, of the occupational therapy profession. Learn to recognize and accept your own limitations—what you or others can and cannot accomplish with clients. Idealism must be balanced with reality. Most experienced practitioners occasionally feel ineffective with some clients. At the same time, you should always put forth your best effort for the benefit and safety of all clients.

Talk It Over With Your Fieldwork Supervisor

Discuss your concerns with your fieldwork supervisor and reflect on your reactions to clients for whom you provide interventions during your fieldwork experience. You may want to ask your supervisor questions like these:

- How do you stay balanced between the real and the ideal?
- How do you balance optimism and hard work with accepting that you will not succeed with every client every time?
- How do you decide which practice and what types of clients will best match your skills as occupational therapy practitioners?

Summary

Developing effective therapeutic relationships is the key to maximizing your effectiveness in helping clients achieve the goals that increase their function, well-being, and quality of life. Remember to meet people where they are and be careful with your own assumptions and biases. Take advantage of the opportunities presented in fieldwork to enhance your abilities to establish therapeutic relationships and practice effective communication skills. At the same time, remember to take care of yourself so you can be of greater help to others.

References

Akhavan, S., & Tillgren, P. (2015). Client/patient perceptions of achieving equity in primary health care: A mixed methods study. *International Journal for Equity in Health, 14*, 65. https://doi.org/10.1186/s12939-015-0196-5

Creel, L., & Yinger, N. (2002). Client-centered quality: Clients' perspectives and barriers to receiving care. *Population Reference Bureau, New Perspectives on Quality Care.* https://www.prb.org/resources/client-centered-quality-clients-perspectives-and-barriers-to-receiving-care/

Ferreira, D. C., Vieira, I., Pedro, M. I., Caldas, P., & Varela, M. (2023). Patient satisfaction with healthcare services and the techniques used for its assessment: A systematic literature review and a bibliometric analysis. *Healthcare (Basel, Switzerland), 11*(5), 639.

Haddad, A., & Doherty, R. (2023). *Health professional and patient interaction* (10th ed.). Saunders.

Sames, K. M. (2015). *Documenting occupational therapy practice* (3rd ed.). Pearson.

Taylor, R. R. (2020). *The intentional relationship: Occupational therapy and use of self* (2nd ed.). F.A. Davis.

PART III.

Client Success Strategies

Chapter 12

When You Finish Your Fieldwork

TOPICS

- Wrapping up your fieldwork rotation
- Registering and preparing for the certification examination
- Applying for a state license

Wrapping Up Your Fieldwork Rotation

At the end of your rotation, you must submit your finalized evaluation forms and requirements to your academic fieldwork coordinator according to your school's process. Make sure you save copies of all documents submitted to the school as part of your clinical passport (see Chapter 1). You may need copies of your final Level II fieldwork evaluations for state licensure boards or transition to another country to practice.

Save your fieldwork documents like you would save copies of your school transcripts. Also, make sure you share a token of appreciation for the mentorship your fieldwork educators provided to you during the last few months of your professional training. Handwritten thank-you notes go a long way!

Registering and Preparing for the Certification Examination

Your academic work and fieldwork experiences are designed to prepare you for the National Board for Certification in Occupational Therapy (NBCOT®) examination. This preparation is similar to reviewing for the SAT or GRE. Multiple options are available to help you review and study for the examination, including books, online training modules, and in-person training sessions. NBCOT and other businesses offer online practice examinations for purchase. Taking practice exams helps you become familiar with the test, identify your weak areas, manage your time while testing, and build confidence. Paying for practice examinations and professional preparation is preferable to having to retake the examination!

The American Occupational Therapy Association (AOTA) offers products for exam preparation:

- AOTA's NBCOT Exam Prep—OTR (https://myaota.aota.org/shop_aota/product/EP_T)
- AOTA's NBCOT Exam Prep—Certified Occupational Therapy Assistant (i.e., COTA®).

Both products include study plans, questions and practice exams, flashcards, and games.

Studying questions and the reasoning behind them helps to understand correct answers. The questions for the certification examination are often written so that several answers are correct, but only one answer is best for the situation described. The study guides and review materials help prepare you for those types of questions. You may have studied during Level II fieldwork, but now is the time to create a structured study schedule and stick to it!

You are responsible for obtaining information and gathering the materials necessary to meet the requirements to sit for the certification exam. Your school may have some information to assist you, but processes can change, so you need to stay current on the most recent information. See NBCOT for details regarding eligibility and the steps from registering and studying to certification.

Registering for this certification exam is your responsibility! In addition to the registration forms and fees, you are also responsible for obtaining transcripts or other supplemental documentation as well as ensuring your college record is accurate and complete for future licensure and NBCOT exam registration. NBCOT requires either a transcript or an official Degree Verification Form from the school confirming that you have passed all requirements for graduation to register for the exam. Once your registration has been officially approved, you will receive an Authorization to Test (ATT) letter from NBCOT that clears you to schedule your examination.

Many students like to check the NBCOT Exam Scoring Calendar to strategically align their test dates with scoring dates so they don't have to wait too long for the results. Ultimately, the best advice is to schedule the exam for when you feel confident and ready to successfully pass it.

NBCOT provides reasonable and appropriate testing accommodations; however, this process can take some time, so it's best to carefully read the Accommodations Handbook on the NBCOT website and follow the steps to apply for accommodations. Before you start Level II fieldwork, meet with your disability support specialists on campus to help you determine what documentation you will need and start the process early. Again, there's no shame in using tools and strategies that work for you. Set yourself up for success! Ensure that you understand the accommodation process and use it to meet your testing needs.

Applying for a State License

It's best to begin preparing for the certification examination and licensing processes before you complete your Level II fieldwork because paperwork and licensing can take longer than you might expect. Students who have not yet passed the NBCOT certification exam can obtain provisional licenses in most states—provided they have proof that they've completed academic and Level II fieldwork requirements. Students usually must show proof of eligibility through college transcripts and/or a copy of the NBCOT ATT letter. A provisional license is valid for a limited time but is typically revoked if the person does not pass the examination on their first attempt following issue of the provisional license. Many students opt to not apply for a provisional license but, rather, wait until they have passed the NBCOT exam before applying for their official state license.

Every licensing board has its own process and procedures. Some may require fingerprinting or background checks for the application. Others may require a letter of reference or character references. In advance of applying for a license, check the licensing board in the state where you plan to practice so you can gather all the necessary documents. Starting early by contacting the licensing board or state occupational therapy association for information can make the difference between starting work soon after completing Level II fieldwork and waiting weeks until your application is processed. Check out AOTA's (n.d.) information on licensure or your specific state's webpage for detailed licensing information.

Keeping the AOTA and state information on licensure close at hand can help you organize the paperwork you will need to complete the certification and licensing processes. An example of how to track licensing information is provided in Exhibit 12.1. You can use the blank form in Exercise 12.1 to track your own information.

Summary

Getting materials together for the certification examination and licensing is the final step toward becoming an occupational therapist or occupational therapy assistant. You will need the information from NBCOT, your state licensing board, and past licensing boards if you move between states or if you have been licensed as an occupational therapy assistant and are now becoming an occupational therapy practitioner. You will need these records for the rest of your professional career—not just as you get started—so keep the documents in a safe place. Your license is often displayed at your workplace, but keep a copy of it with your important papers. Scan and retain electronic copies of all these records as well.

Remember that your friendly faculty members—your academic fieldwork coordinator and teachers—are available and want to support you throughout your journey from graduation to licensure. They would be more than happy to answer questions and help you find the resources you need.

Congratulations on finishing Level II fieldwork and joining the profession as an occupational therapy practitioner! Welcome!

EXHIBIT 12.1. Tracking Licensing Information: An Example

Licensing Item	Examples of How to Track Licensing Information
State from which I have requested information: *California*	Address, phone, and fax number of licensing board: *California Board of OT, 444 N. 3rd St., Suite 444, Sacramento, CA 95814*
Required documents (specific from state to state): • *Fingerprints with background check* • *Official transcripts* • *Letter of moral character* • *NBCOT® ATT letter or official certification results*	Date completed or requested: • *Completed May 24* • *Requested June 1* • *Mailed June 16* • *Requested June 20*

Note. NBCOT® = National Board for Certification in Occupational Therapy; ATT = Authorization to Test.

Exercise 12.1. **Tracking Your Licensing Information**

Licensing Item	Examples of How to Track Licensing Information
State from which I have requested information:	Address, phone, and fax number of licensing board:
Required documents (specific from state to state):	Date completed or requested:

Reference

American Occupational Therapy Association. (n.d.). *Licensure.* https://www.aota.org/career/state-licensure

Chapter 13

Tracking Clients

TOPICS

- Your client-tracking tool kit
- How to keep track of your clients
- Common sources of client information
- Keeping client information confidential
- Meetings and documentation timelines

I've worked with a few therapists who were wonderful with clients in face-to-face sessions but didn't keep up with documentation and all the other things that need to be done so we can keep seeing clients, providing therapy, and making a difference in people's lives. Our department can't afford those people. There are so many demands on our time, and we don't get paid without good documentation.

Sometimes, it seems sad that someone who makes the client feel so good is a liability to the department, but the reality is that if we don't keep track of our clients and do accurate and timely documentation, nobody will get paid, and the entire department receives closer scrutiny, resulting in slower reimbursement. We may love our work for what it does for people, but we also want a paycheck.

—Occupational therapy supervisor
commenting on the reality of the clinic

As a student, you may have kept track of assignments, examinations, and papers using a digital or paper calendar and by making lists of when things were due. Similar systems are valuable in the clinic for the rest of your professional career. You will have more flexibility regarding some calendar items and less flexibility in others. You no longer have grades or professors to keep your attention to task. Now, you have responsibilities to clients, insurance companies or other reimbursing agencies, physicians, and fellow workers. Find a system that works for you, whether it's using colored pens, sticky tabs, apps, or other techniques. While you are still a student and reporting to your clinical fieldwork supervisor, demonstrating that you are organized will project a positive impression and save time for other questions and client issues that need to be discussed.

You won't be able to fit all the information you have about a client in the treatment record, nor should you. The purpose of some information is to provide you with reminders. This type of information typically does not need to be available to others who read the treatment record. For example, although you would document how a client scored overall on a particular assessment along with your interpretation of the client's performance, the scoring form for the assessment would generally not be part of the client's record. You would retain the scoring form for comparison the next time you evaluated the client.

Your Client-Tracking Tool Kit

Your tools for keeping track of your clients are similar to those you used as a student to track assignments, examinations, and papers. However, your system needs to make sense to other individuals who will rely on it in case you need someone to cover your clients. The focus is on client needs rather than your individual needs. If another occupational therapy practitioner needs to cover your clients, if you are out sick, or if you share client coverage as a result of scheduling, your system has to make sense to your peers.

When tracking your clients, you will have two big items. First, you will have individual client folders (hard copy or digital) that you have created—not the legal record of client treatment, although your own records can be subpoenaed. Second, you will need to create a central tracking sheet of all your clients in addition to your own personal calendar.

Client Folders

Identify clients only by their initials or another anonymous way to maintain confidentiality. Use digital or paper folders to store memos from client conferences, forms from assessments, and notes to yourself about treatment ideas that might work with a particular client. Creative therapy ideas don't always occur at convenient times, so when you have an idea, you can drop a note to yourself in the folder. These items will help trigger information that may need to go into documentation, but, for various reasons, they might be unnecessary or unsuitable for any record except your working folder.

Tracking Sheets

A *tracking sheet* is a tool used to document and monitor a client's progress, skills, and performance in specific areas so you can track interventions and, if necessary, adjust your approach. First, you need to list all the information, meetings, or documentation events that should go on your calendar. With this list, you can check off the necessary items and make sure to look at a note, communication, meeting, or other deadline that needs to be met for clients in the clinical setting. Examples of the types of information needed for a tracking sheet are listed in Exhibit 13.1.

EXHIBIT 13.1. What to Track on Your Tracking Sheet

Typically, you need to track and mark on your calendar the following types of client meetings and commonly required documentation:

- initial note within 24 hours of admission and/or first assessment session
- full evaluation (sometimes the same as initial note); varies, but usually is done within 48 hours of admission and/or beginning assessment
- documentation in relation to frequency of sessions: daily, weekly, and so on
- team conferences related to client issues or progress
- summaries as required by the agency: weekly, monthly, and so on
- family conferences or team meetings with client and/or family present
- discharge summaries

You can organize materials in many ways, including the one presented in Exhibit 13.2, which shows an example week. (A blank copy of this form as well as other helpful tools, such as calendar pages, are included in Part V of this book.) Post a form like the one illustrated in Exhibit 13.2 in your workspace or carry it on a clipboard for easy access.

Let's consider how to use this tool. Looking at the example in Exhibit 13.2, say today's date is June 16. By glancing at the form, the occupational therapy practitioner knows that they will have three team conferences today and three summary reports due tomorrow, June 17. Proactive planning like this will help you keep on top of your responsibilities. The important thing is to have everything you need to know about every client centralized and available at a glance.

Ask other students how they keep organized and see whether your professors or fieldwork supervisors will share their tips and techniques to track and schedule events, due dates, meetings, and other responsibilities. Making an accurate schedule of your responsibilities is an essential skill of successful occupational therapy practitioners. It can make the difference between being reactive and proactive and even enable you to look calm to clients and peers when you are tightly scheduled.

Be like the duck: calm on the surface and paddling like crazy under the water!

Talk It Over With Your Fieldwork Supervisor

Ask your fieldwork supervisor for additional guidance in creating a tracking sheet that works in their particular setting. Have they found something particularly effective related to their setting, or can they offer general tips for organizing clinical information?

EXHIBIT 13.2. Sample Tracking Sheet

Crossing out (never erasing) events help you track completion of tasks.						
Date	**Day**	**Client 1: Sam**	**Client 2: Suzette**	**Client 3: Fred**	**Client 4: Alicia**	**Client 5: Jorge**
June 1	W					
June 2	T		Admitted initial note			
June 3	F	Admitted initial note				
June 4/5	S/S	Not scheduled to work; leave suggestions for weekend therapists				
June 5	S					
June 6	M	Full eval report due	Full eval report due			
June 7	Tu			Admitted initial note	Admitted initial note	
June 8	W					
June 9	Th			Team conf	Team conf	
June 10	F			Weekly summary	Weekly summary	Weekly summary
June 11/12	S/S	Not scheduled to work; leave suggestions for weekend therapists				
June 13	M					
June 14	Tu	Team conf	Team conf			Full eval due
June 15	W	Weekly summary	Weekly summary			
June 16	Th			Team conf	Team conf	
June 17	F		Proposed discharge (summary)	Weekly summary	Weekly summary	
June 18/19	S/S	Scheduled to work weekend coverage				
June 20	M					Proposed discharge (summary)

Note. M = Monday; Tu = Tuesday; W = Wednesday; Th = Thursday; F = Friday; S/S = Saturday/Sunday; eval = evaluation; conf = conference.
Consider other abbreviations of your own, but always note what your abbreviations mean so you don't forget them. Remember that abbreviations you make up cannot be used in documentation!

How to Keep Track of Your Clients

In addition to documentation deadlines, you need accurate client data at your fingertips without requiring the client's official legal record or chart, which may be unavailable when you need information. Summarizing information on your own tracking sheet makes it easier to refresh your memory with a particular client (see Exhibit 13.3).

Make the most of your records by keeping a list of the key information you will need as a client's occupational therapy practitioner. Many practitioners keep a copy of their evaluation and summary notes for this purpose. Your own client information sheet also allows you to review key information when you are working on creative ways to meet your client's goals. Some of the information you want in your client file will come from team reports in the legal record or referral.

EXHIBIT 13.3. Documentation and Report Tracking Sheet

- A tracking sheet does not have to be fancy to be effective.
- Photocopy this page or design your own.
- When listing events, use colors to denote particular responsibilities.
- For your own record of completion and to give you a sense of what you have accomplished, cross out tasks that are done.

Date/Day	Client 1	Client 2	Client 3	Client 4	Client 5

Common Sources of Client Information

Client information comes from formal and informal sources. In most settings, the primary information comes from the client's chart or referral forms you receive when you initiate treatment. Other information comes from informal discussions with family members, who may provide important insights regarding the kind and level of support the client has available to them outside of the clinical setting. You may also learn about the client's interests, which may help you motivate their involvement in therapy sessions. Important information can be communicated in casual conversations with clients, friends, family, or others with whom the client interacts, but listen carefully to separate gossip from data. Check your information before acting on it!

Keeping Client Information Confidential

Some clients do not want it known that they are receiving therapy. Most don't mind, but the confidentiality of all clients is important. In some locations, you may even be providing treatment to people who are registered under aliases. Most of the time, confidentiality simply involves respect and keeping someone's personal business private, and it is a legal requirement.

In addition to using short names or initials when you make notes about specific clients, remember that conversations can be overheard. Keep client names confidential unless you know you are discussing them in a secure location. You never know when a relative or friend, or someone who knows the person but shouldn't know their personal information, may be within earshot. Err on the side of caution!

Meetings and Documentation Timelines

Before you start using the client tracking sheets provided in this book, be sure you know your clinical site's information, regular meetings, documentation requirements, and so on. Make a list of all of your anticipated meetings and documentation responsibilities.

After compiling your list, review it with your clinical fieldwork supervisor to be sure you have recorded all the items. The list will vary from agency to agency depending on whether the clients are receiving therapy in the community, whether they are receiving therapy as inpatients or outpatients, the frequency with which you see your clients, third-party payer requirements, and so on. See Exhibit 13.4 for a sample list of meetings regularly required at clinical sites. Make a similar list of the meetings you need to track in your fieldwork setting. Use the calendar in Part V of this book to mark down meetings and documentation responsibilities—just as you have done with your academic work.

EXHIBIT 13.4. Examples of Customary Meetings Required at Clinical Sites

Meeting	Frequency	Schedule (Specific Dates)
Client rounds	Weekly	Tu at 9 a.m.
Occupational therapy meetings	Biweekly	F at 8 a.m.
Team meetings	Weekly	W at 12:30 p.m.
Discharge conferences	As needed	
Family conferences	As needed	
Meetings with fieldwork supervisor	Weekly	M at 3:30 p.m. and F at 12:30 p.m.
[Other meetings]		

Note. M = Monday; Tu = Tuesday; W = Wednesday; F = Friday.

Summary

Confidentially tracking client information will help you provide effective client interventions, enhance preparation for sessions with clients and meetings with peers, and keep you up-to-date on the progress and needs of your clients. Likewise, keeping a list or calendar of administrative meetings and documentation deadlines will help ensure you do not miss these essential tasks. The sample forms in this chapter are designed to help you organize them. An organized calendar not only helps decrease stress at work and home but can help a clinician with a busy schedule minimize the hassles of scheduling and maximize their focus on the client.

PART IV.

Keeping It All Together: Survival Data for Each of Your Level II Fieldwork Experiences

Chapter 14

Tracking Information: First Level II Fieldwork

TOPICS

- Making the most of what's in this chapter
- Levels of competence related to clinical skills development and need for supervision

TOOLS

- How Do I Respond to Feedback? (Chapter 2)
- Identifying Good Goals (Chapter 3)
- Writing Professional Goals (Chapter 3)
- Compilation of Necessary Fieldwork Information: At-a-Glance Checklist (Chapter 4)
- Levels of Competence Related to Clinical Skills and Need for Supervision (Chapter 7)
- Gathering Information on a Team Before Joining (Chapter 8)
- Frames of Reference and Fieldwork Sites (Chapter 9)
- Fundamental Elements of Documentation (Chapter 10)
- Learning by Example: Well-Written Documentation (Chapter 10)
- Documentation and Report Tracking Sheet (Chapter 13)
- Calendar

Making the Most of What's in This Chapter

This part of the book consists of two chapters—this one on the first Level II fieldwork and Chapter 15 on the second Level II fieldwork. Both chapters contain some of the same tools (e.g., exercises, exhibits) that were presented to you in earlier chapters, which explained how these tools can be helpful. For easy reference, a list is provided at the beginning of both chapters that includes the title of each resource and the chapter in which it first appears. In addition, this chapter introduces the Sample Tracking Sheet and calendar pages.

The tools are grouped and repeated here so you can keep all the information relevant to each fieldwork site in one location in this survival guide and so that you have this information appearing immediately before your daily calendar pages. Consider using sticky notes to help the resource on which you are focusing stand out. Use the same technique to denote the current day in the daily calendar pages. Completing the exercises or forms before or in the first week of your clinical assignments can help you be more organized and informed at your fieldwork sites.

Levels of Competence Related to Clinical Skills Development and Need for Supervision

Remember: There is no usual or customary amount of time that one spends in each level of supervision. For some clinicians, it may take twice as long as others to achieve general supervision levels, and there are some good clinicians who remain most comfortable with routine or general supervision throughout their careers.

Part of what this process can help you identify is the type of setting where you will be most comfortable practicing. Working on a team that includes other occupational therapy practitioners offers opportunities for collaboration for some and general supervision for others. Working in home health settings requires a clinician who has achieved at least minimal supervision because that clinician will be working in constantly changing environments (e.g., clients' homes) with constantly changing groups of individuals (e.g., clients, members of the community) and will need to carry with them assessments and other items that can contribute to an effective intervention. Use your fieldwork time to learn, observe, and strengthen your skills so that you are prepared for entry-level practice and have gained an awareness of the type of clinical setting in which you want to work and can flourish as a clinician.

How Do I Respond to Feedback?

Evaluate your response to feedback (see Figure 2.1). On the lines below, state the problem or issue about which you are concerned and describe it as concretely as you can. Putting thoughts in writing can be a powerful way to be introspective and clarify what you want to communicate.

____

____

____

____

Then, using the grid that follows, indicate how positively you see yourself at this moment for each item listed.

Where Do You See Yourself Today?

Positive	++	+	?	–	– –	Negative
Actively listen						Am defensive, ignore
Envision or create opportunity, be open						Am resentful
Understand and clarify						Don't listen, don't grow
Engage in introspective review						Ignore feedback
Do it better next time						Do it the same again and again
Have good self-esteem, see growth toward becoming clinician						Have poor self-esteem, ignore a chance to grow

Note. ++ = very positive; + = positive; ? = unsure; – = negative; – – = very negative.

Next, answer the following eight questions:

1. What can I do to change how I view and communicate the problem?

2. Do I need to listen more carefully to the content rather than react to the tone? What might I be ignoring?

3. Is this an opportunity for me to change and become a better clinician?

4. What can I do to deal effectively with this situation?

5. If I need to confront someone, how can I phrase it so that I do not increase my own or the other person's defensiveness? *Write out variations of what may be said.*

6. How could I review the situation and avoid being hypersensitive about comments that could have a different meaning than what I thought I understood?

7. Have I asked a significant, unbiased person (e.g., not my best friend who always agrees with me) about other ways to interpret the situation?

8. After dealing with the situation, what were the best approaches I used and why? What are the approaches I should avoid, and why?

Best approaches	**Why are these "best approaches"?**
Approaches I should avoid:	**Why should I avoid these approaches?**

Identifying Good Goals

For each of the following goals, decide if it meets the RUMBA requirements. In Columns 2 through 6, put a check mark when a goal meets the measurability requirement and a zero (0) when the goal does not. Then revise each of the goals that does not meet all of the RUMBA requirements.

Goal	Relevant	Understandable	Measurable	Behavioral	Achievable
1. Arrive at work every day on time.					
2. Achieve the highest rating on most of my evaluations.					
3. Improve my ability to evaluate clients.					
4. By the end of next week, learn 5 new activities to use when working with stroke clients.					
5. Improve the accuracy of my documentation.					

The following is my revision of each goal so that it meets all of the RUMBA requirements:

1. ______________________________

____

2. ______________________________

____

3. ______________________________

____

4. ______________________________

____

5. ______________________________

____

Writing Professional Goals

Write two professional goals that you want to achieve during fieldwork. In Columns 2 through 6, briefly describe how each goal meets each of the RUMBA requirements.

Professional Goal 1	Reasonable	Understand-able	Measurable	Behavioral	Achievable
Professional Goal 2	**Reasonable**	**Understand-able**	**Measurable**	**Behavioral**	**Achievable**

Compilation of Necessary Fieldwork Information: At-a-Glance Checklist

Item	Location of Item	Comments
Supplies (consumables)		
Equipment and storage		
Forms		
Policy and procedure manuals		
Instructions for equipment		
Library and location of resource materials		
Other necessary items or information		

Levels of Competence Related to Clinical Skills and Need for Supervision

Level	Distinction	Guiding Principle	Type of Supervision Needed	Date Achieved
Novice Can follow basic rules	No distinctions between rules and context in which the rules are applied	Basic rules and procedures	Close	
Advanced beginner Can assess and adapt to deviations from rules and procedures	Actions dictated by rules versus actions dictated by situation	Important aspects of a situation	Close	
Competent entry-level practitioner Can assess and adapt to important aspects of a situation	Actions dictated by situation versus actions dictated by general plan	General principles	Routine	
Proficient professional Can assess and adapt to deviations from plan	Actuals dictated by general plan versus actions dictated by intuition	Patterns and scenarios	General	
Expert Can assess and adapt to deviations from a pattern; can focus on critical factors	Actions and situations are synonymous	Holistic, integrated images and intuition	Minimal	Not achievable during fieldwork

Gathering Information on a Team Before Joining

Agency or site name:
Type of team (i.e., focus, disciplines, purpose):
Purpose of the team:
Team goals or priorities (i.e., how the team knows if its work is completed):
Members or disciplines represented on the team:
• What would be my responsibilities as a member of the team?
• What would I need to know to carry out my team responsibilities?
• Where could I get help if I needed it?
• What skills would I be bringing to the team?
• How could I demonstrate support of other team members?

• What else could I do to help the team produce results and achieve its goals?
• What would I be expected to prepare and bring to team meetings?
• What else would I need to do or prepare for work on this particular team?

Frames of Reference and Fieldwork Sites

Fieldwork or clinical site:	Frame(s) of reference:
Types of clients (i.e., diagnoses or reason for referral):	How this frame of reference is applied with clients:
What would be common goals for intervention related to this frame of reference in this particular setting?	What other influences does this frame of reference have in this particular setting?

Fundamental Elements of Documentation

- Client's full name and case number on each page of documentation
- Date and type of occupational therapy contact
- Identification of type of documentation, agency, and department name
- Occupational therapy signature with first name or initial, last name, and professional designation
- When applicable on notes or reports, signature of the recorder directly at the end of the note without space left between the body of the note and the signature
- Countersignature by an occupational therapist on documentation written by students or occupational therapy assistants when required by law or by the facility
- Acceptable terminology defined within the boundaries of the setting
- Abbreviation usage as acceptable within the boundaries of the setting
- When no facility requirements are listed, errors are corrected by drawing a single line through an error and initialing the correction; correction fluid or tape and erasures are not acceptable
- Adherence to professional standards of terminology used to document occupational therapy
- Disposal of records within law and agency requirements
- Compliance with confidentiality standards
- Compliance with legal and agency requirements of storage of records

Learning by Example: Well-Written Documentation

Ask your supervisor to provide examples of well-written documentation specific to the site where you are doing your fieldwork. Then analyze the way that content is presented. What you'll be doing here is similar to completing chart reviews, as is done in every health care facility.

• What makes the documentation easy to read and understand?
• How does the writer include important information without being too wordy?
• What type of information is included in each section of the documentation?

Documentation and Report Tracking Sheet

- A tracking sheet does not have to be fancy to be effective.
- Photocopy this page or design your own.
- When listing events, use colors to denote particular responsibilities.
- For your own record of completion and to give you a sense of what you have accomplished, cross out tasks that are done.

Date/Day	Client 1	Client 2	Client 3	Client 4	Client 5

Calendar

Tasks	Tasks

Day/Date	HOURLY APPOINTMENT SCHEDULE	Day/Date
6 AM		6 AM
7 AM		7 AM
8 AM		8 AM
9 AM		9 AM
10 AM		10 AM
11 AM		11 AM
12 PM		12 PM
1 PM		1 PM
2 PM		2 PM
3 PM		3 PM
4 PM		4 PM
5 PM		5 PM
6 PM		6 PM

Notes:

Calendar

Tasks	**Tasks**

Day/Date	**HOURLY APPOINTMENT SCHEDULE**	**Day/Date**

6 AM ______	6 AM ______
7 AM ______	7 AM ______
8 AM ______	8 AM ______
9 AM ______	9 AM ______
10 AM ______	10 AM ______
11 AM ______	11 AM ______
12 PM ______	12 PM ______
1 PM ______	1 PM ______
2 PM ______	2 PM ______
3 PM ______	3 PM ______
4 PM ______	4 PM ______
5 PM ______	5 PM ______
6 PM ______	6 PM ______

Notes:

Calendar

Tasks	Tasks

Day/Date	HOURLY APPOINTMENT SCHEDULE	Day/Date

6 AM	6 AM
7 AM	7 AM
8 AM	8 AM
9 AM	9 AM
10 AM	10 AM
11 AM	11 AM
12 PM	12 PM
1 PM	1 PM
2 PM	2 PM
3 PM	3 PM
4 PM	4 PM
5 PM	5 PM
6 PM	6 PM

Notes:

Calendar

Tasks	**Tasks**

Day/Date	**HOURLY APPOINTMENT SCHEDULE**	**Day/Date**

6 AM	6 AM
7 AM	7 AM
8 AM	8 AM
9 AM	9 AM
10 AM	10 AM
11 AM	11 AM
12 PM	12 PM
1 PM	1 PM
2 PM	2 PM
3 PM	3 PM
4 PM	4 PM
5 PM	5 PM
6 PM	6 PM

Notes:

Calendar

Tasks	Tasks

Day/Date	HOURLY APPOINTMENT SCHEDULE	Day/Date

6 AM	6 AM
7 AM	7 AM
8 AM	8 AM
9 AM	9 AM
10 AM	10 AM
11 AM	11 AM
12 PM	12 PM
1 PM	1 PM
2 PM	2 PM
3 PM	3 PM
4 PM	4 PM
5 PM	5 PM
6 PM	6 PM

Notes:

Calendar

Tasks	Tasks

Day/Date	HOURLY APPOINTMENT SCHEDULE	Day/Date
6 AM		6 AM
7 AM		7 AM
8 AM		8 AM
9 AM		9 AM
10 AM		10 AM
11 AM		11 AM
12 PM		12 PM
1 PM		1 PM
2 PM		2 PM
3 PM		3 PM
4 PM		4 PM
5 PM		5 PM
6 PM		6 PM

Notes:

Calendar

Tasks	Tasks

Day/Date	HOURLY APPOINTMENT SCHEDULE	Day/Date

6 AM	6 AM
7 AM	7 AM
8 AM	8 AM
9 AM	9 AM
10 AM	10 AM
11 AM	11 AM
12 PM	12 PM
1 PM	1 PM
2 PM	2 PM
3 PM	3 PM
4 PM	4 PM
5 PM	5 PM
6 PM	6 PM

Notes:

Calendar

Tasks	**Tasks**

Day/Date	**HOURLY APPOINTMENT SCHEDULE**	**Day/Date**

6 AM	6 AM
7 AM	7 AM
8 AM	8 AM
9 AM	9 AM
10 AM	10 AM
11 AM	11 AM
12 PM	12 PM
1 PM	1 PM
2 PM	2 PM
3 PM	3 PM
4 PM	4 PM
5 PM	5 PM
6 PM	6 PM

Notes:

Calendar

Tasks		Tasks
Day/Date	**HOURLY APPOINTMENT SCHEDULE**	**Day/Date**
6 AM		6 AM
7 AM		7 AM
8 AM		8 AM
9 AM		9 AM
10 AM		10 AM
11 AM		11 AM
12 PM		12 PM
1 PM		1 PM
2 PM		2 PM
3 PM		3 PM
4 PM		4 PM
5 PM		5 PM
6 PM		6 PM

Notes:

Calendar

Tasks	Tasks

Day/Date	HOURLY APPOINTMENT SCHEDULE	Day/Date

6 AM ______	6 AM ______
7 AM ______	7 AM ______
8 AM ______	8 AM ______
9 AM ______	9 AM ______
10 AM ______	10 AM ______
11 AM ______	11 AM ______
12 PM ______	12 PM ______
1 PM ______	1 PM ______
2 PM ______	2 PM ______
3 PM ______	3 PM ______
4 PM ______	4 PM ______
5 PM ______	5 PM ______
6 PM ______	6 PM ______

Notes:

Calendar

Tasks	Tasks

Day/Date	HOURLY APPOINTMENT SCHEDULE	Day/Date

6 AM	6 AM
7 AM	7 AM
8 AM	8 AM
9 AM	9 AM
10 AM	10 AM
11 AM	11 AM
12 PM	12 PM
1 PM	1 PM
2 PM	2 PM
3 PM	3 PM
4 PM	4 PM
5 PM	5 PM
6 PM	6 PM

Notes:

Calendar

Tasks	**Tasks**

Day/Date	**HOURLY APPOINTMENT SCHEDULE**	**Day/Date**

6 AM	6 AM
7 AM	7 AM
8 AM	8 AM
9 AM	9 AM
10 AM	10 AM
11 AM	11 AM
12 PM	12 PM
1 PM	1 PM
2 PM	2 PM
3 PM	3 PM
4 PM	4 PM
5 PM	5 PM
6 PM	6 PM

Notes:

Calendar

Tasks	Tasks

Day/Date	HOURLY APPOINTMENT SCHEDULE	Day/Date
6 AM		6 AM
7 AM		7 AM
8 AM		8 AM
9 AM		9 AM
10 AM		10 AM
11 AM		11 AM
12 PM		12 PM
1 PM		1 PM
2 PM		2 PM
3 PM		3 PM
4 PM		4 PM
5 PM		5 PM
6 PM		6 PM

Notes:

Calendar

Tasks	Tasks

Day/Date	HOURLY APPOINTMENT SCHEDULE	Day/Date

6 AM	6 AM
7 AM	7 AM
8 AM	8 AM
9 AM	9 AM
10 AM	10 AM
11 AM	11 AM
12 PM	12 PM
1 PM	1 PM
2 PM	2 PM
3 PM	3 PM
4 PM	4 PM
5 PM	5 PM
6 PM	6 PM

Notes:

Calendar

Tasks	Tasks

Day/Date	HOURLY APPOINTMENT SCHEDULE	Day/Date
6 AM		6 AM
7 AM		7 AM
8 AM		8 AM
9 AM		9 AM
10 AM		10 AM
11 AM		11 AM
12 PM		12 PM
1 PM		1 PM
2 PM		2 PM
3 PM		3 PM
4 PM		4 PM
5 PM		5 PM
6 PM		6 PM

Notes:

Calendar

Tasks	Tasks

Day/Date	HOURLY APPOINTMENT SCHEDULE	Day/Date

6 AM	6 AM
7 AM	7 AM
8 AM	8 AM
9 AM	9 AM
10 AM	10 AM
11 AM	11 AM
12 PM	12 PM
1 PM	1 PM
2 PM	2 PM
3 PM	3 PM
4 PM	4 PM
5 PM	5 PM
6 PM	6 PM

Notes:

Calendar

Tasks	Tasks

Day/Date	HOURLY APPOINTMENT SCHEDULE	Day/Date

6 AM ______	6 AM ______
7 AM ______	7 AM ______
8 AM ______	8 AM ______
9 AM ______	9 AM ______
10 AM ______	10 AM ______
11 AM ______	11 AM ______
12 PM ______	12 PM ______
1 PM ______	1 PM ______
2 PM ______	2 PM ______
3 PM ______	3 PM ______
4 PM ______	4 PM ______
5 PM ______	5 PM ______
6 PM ______	6 PM ______

Notes:

Calendar

Tasks	**Tasks**

Day/Date	**HOURLY APPOINTMENT SCHEDULE**	**Day/Date**

6 AM	6 AM
7 AM	7 AM
8 AM	8 AM
9 AM	9 AM
10 AM	10 AM
11 AM	11 AM
12 PM	12 PM
1 PM	1 PM
2 PM	2 PM
3 PM	3 PM
4 PM	4 PM
5 PM	5 PM
6 PM	6 PM

Notes:

Calendar

Tasks	**Tasks**

Day/Date	HOURLY APPOINTMENT SCHEDULE	Day/Date

6 AM	6 AM
7 AM	7 AM
8 AM	8 AM
9 AM	9 AM
10 AM	10 AM
11 AM	11 AM
12 PM	12 PM
1 PM	1 PM
2 PM	2 PM
3 PM	3 PM
4 PM	4 PM
5 PM	5 PM
6 PM	6 PM

Notes:

Calendar

Tasks	Tasks

Day/Date	HOURLY APPOINTMENT SCHEDULE	Day/Date

6 AM	6 AM
7 AM	7 AM
8 AM	8 AM
9 AM	9 AM
10 AM	10 AM
11 AM	11 AM
12 PM	12 PM
1 PM	1 PM
2 PM	2 PM
3 PM	3 PM
4 PM	4 PM
5 PM	5 PM
6 PM	6 PM

Notes:

Calendar

Tasks	Tasks

Day/Date	HOURLY APPOINTMENT SCHEDULE	Day/Date

6 AM	6 AM
7 AM	7 AM
8 AM	8 AM
9 AM	9 AM
10 AM	10 AM
11 AM	11 AM
12 PM	12 PM
1 PM	1 PM
2 PM	2 PM
3 PM	3 PM
4 PM	4 PM
5 PM	5 PM
6 PM	6 PM

Notes:

Calendar

Tasks	Tasks

Day/Date	HOURLY APPOINTMENT SCHEDULE	Day/Date

6 AM	6 AM
7 AM	7 AM
8 AM	8 AM
9 AM	9 AM
10 AM	10 AM
11 AM	11 AM
12 PM	12 PM
1 PM	1 PM
2 PM	2 PM
3 PM	3 PM
4 PM	4 PM
5 PM	5 PM
6 PM	6 PM

Notes:

Calendar

Tasks	Tasks

Day/Date	HOURLY APPOINTMENT SCHEDULE	Day/Date

6 AM	6 AM
7 AM	7 AM
8 AM	8 AM
9 AM	9 AM
10 AM	10 AM
11 AM	11 AM
12 PM	12 PM
1 PM	1 PM
2 PM	2 PM
3 PM	3 PM
4 PM	4 PM
5 PM	5 PM
6 PM	6 PM

Notes:

Calendar

Tasks	Tasks

Day/Date	HOURLY APPOINTMENT SCHEDULE	Day/Date

6 AM	6 AM
7 AM	7 AM
8 AM	8 AM
9 AM	9 AM
10 AM	10 AM
11 AM	11 AM
12 PM	12 PM
1 PM	1 PM
2 PM	2 PM
3 PM	3 PM
4 PM	4 PM
5 PM	5 PM
6 PM	6 PM

Notes:

Calendar

Tasks	Tasks

Day/Date	HOURLY APPOINTMENT SCHEDULE	Day/Date

6 AM	6 AM
7 AM	7 AM
8 AM	8 AM
9 AM	9 AM
10 AM	10 AM
11 AM	11 AM
12 PM	12 PM
1 PM	1 PM
2 PM	2 PM
3 PM	3 PM
4 PM	4 PM
5 PM	5 PM
6 PM	6 PM

Notes:

Calendar

Tasks	**Tasks**

Day/Date	**HOURLY APPOINTMENT SCHEDULE**	**Day/Date**

6 AM	6 AM
7 AM	7 AM
8 AM	8 AM
9 AM	9 AM
10 AM	10 AM
11 AM	11 AM
12 PM	12 PM
1 PM	1 PM
2 PM	2 PM
3 PM	3 PM
4 PM	4 PM
5 PM	5 PM
6 PM	6 PM

Notes:

Calendar

Tasks	Tasks

Day/Date	HOURLY APPOINTMENT SCHEDULE	Day/Date

6 AM	6 AM
7 AM	7 AM
8 AM	8 AM
9 AM	9 AM
10 AM	10 AM
11 AM	11 AM
12 PM	12 PM
1 PM	1 PM
2 PM	2 PM
3 PM	3 PM
4 PM	4 PM
5 PM	5 PM
6 PM	6 PM

Notes:

Calendar

Tasks	Tasks

Day/Date	HOURLY APPOINTMENT SCHEDULE	Day/Date
6 AM		6 AM
7 AM		7 AM
8 AM		8 AM
9 AM		9 AM
10 AM		10 AM
11 AM		11 AM
12 PM		12 PM
1 PM		1 PM
2 PM		2 PM
3 PM		3 PM
4 PM		4 PM
5 PM		5 PM
6 PM		6 PM

Notes:

Calendar

Tasks	Tasks

Day/Date	HOURLY APPOINTMENT SCHEDULE	Day/Date
6 AM		6 AM
7 AM		7 AM
8 AM		8 AM
9 AM		9 AM
10 AM		10 AM
11 AM		11 AM
12 PM		12 PM
1 PM		1 PM
2 PM		2 PM
3 PM		3 PM
4 PM		4 PM
5 PM		5 PM
6 PM		6 PM

Notes:

Calendar

Tasks	**Tasks**

Day/Date	**HOURLY APPOINTMENT SCHEDULE**	**Day/Date**

6 AM	6 AM
7 AM	7 AM
8 AM	8 AM
9 AM	9 AM
10 AM	10 AM
11 AM	11 AM
12 PM	12 PM
1 PM	1 PM
2 PM	2 PM
3 PM	3 PM
4 PM	4 PM
5 PM	5 PM
6 PM	6 PM

Notes:

Chapter 15

Tracking Information: Second Level II Fieldwork

TOPICS

- Making the most of what's in this chapter
- Levels of competence related to clinical skills development and need for supervision

TOOLS

- How Do I Respond to Feedback? (Chapter 2)
- Identifying Good Goals (Chapter 3)
- Writing Professional Goals (Chapter 3)
- Compilation of Necessary Fieldwork Information: At-a-Glance Checklist (Chapter 4)
- Levels of Competence Related to Clinical Skills and Need for Supervision (Chapter 7)
- Gathering Information on a Team Before Joining (Chapter 8)
- Frames of Reference and Fieldwork Sites (Chapter 9)
- Fundamental Elements of Documentation (Chapter 10)
- Learning by Example: Well-Written Documentation (Chapter 10)
- Documentation and Report Tracking Sheet (Chapter 13)
- Calendar

Making the Most of What's in This Chapter

Like Chapter 14, this chapter contains some of the same tools that were presented to you in earlier chapters, which explained how these tools could be helpful. For easy reference, a list is provided at the beginning of both chapters that includes the title of each resource and the chapter in which it first appears.

The tools are grouped and repeated in this chapter so you can keep all the information relevant to each fieldwork site in one location in this survival guide and so that you have this information appearing immediately before your daily calendar pages. Consider using sticky notes to help the resource on which you are focusing stand out. Use the same technique to denote the current day in the daily calendar pages. Completing the exercises or forms before or in the first week of your clinical assignments can help you be more organized and informed at your fieldwork sites.

Levels of Competence Related to Clinical Skills Development and Need for Supervision

Remember: There is no usual or customary amount of time that one spends in each level of supervision. For some clinicians, it may take twice as long as others to achieve general supervision levels, and there are some good clinicians who remain most comfortable with routine or general supervision throughout their careers.

Part of what this process can help you identify is the type of setting where you will be most comfortable practicing. Working on a team that includes other occupational therapy practitioners offers opportunities for collaboration for some and general supervision for others. Working in home health settings requires a clinician who has achieved at least minimal supervision because that clinician will be working in constantly changing environments (e.g., clients' homes) with constantly changing groups of individuals (e.g., clients, members of the community) and will need to carry with them assessments and other items that can contribute to an effective intervention. Use your fieldwork time to learn, observe, and strengthen your skills so that you are prepared both for entry-level practice and have gained an awareness of the type of clinical setting in which you want to work and can flourish as a clinician.

How Do I Respond to Feedback?

Evaluate your response to feedback (see Figure 2.1). On the lines below, state the problem or issue about which you are concerned and describe it as concretely as you can. Putting thoughts in writing can be a powerful way to be introspective and clarify what you want to communicate.

____

____

____

____

Then, using the grid that follows, indicate how positively you see yourself at this moment for each item listed.

Where Do You See Yourself Today?

Positive	++	+	?	–	– –	Negative
Actively listen						Am defensive, ignore
Envision or create opportunity, be open						Am resentful
Understand and clarify						Don't listen, don't grow
Engage in introspective review						Ignore feedback
Do it better next time						Do it the same again and again
Have good self-esteem, see growth toward becoming clinician						Have poor self-esteem, ignore a chance to grow

Note. ++ = very positive; + = positive; ? = unsure; – = negative; – – = very negative.

Next, answer the following eight questions:

1. What can I do to change how I view and communicate the problem?

____

____

____

____

2. Do I need to listen more carefully to the content rather than react to the tone? What might I be ignoring?

____

____

____

____

3. Is this an opportunity for me to change and become a better clinician?

____

____

____

____

4. What can I do to deal effectively with this situation?

____

____

____

____

5. If I need to confront someone, how can I phrase it so that I do not increase my own or the other person's defensiveness? *Write out variations of what may be said.*

____

____

____

____

6. How could I review the situation and avoid being hypersensitive about comments that could have a different meaning than what I thought I understood?

____

____

____

____

7. Have I asked a significant, unbiased person (e.g., not my best friend who always agrees with me) about other ways to interpret the situation?

____

____

____

____

8. After dealing with the situation, what were the best approaches I used and why? What are the approaches I should avoid, and why?

Best approaches	**Why are these "best approaches"?**
Approaches I should avoid:	**Why should I avoid these approaches?**

Identifying Good Goals

For each of the following goals, decide if it meets the RUMBA requirements. In Columns 2 through 6, put a check mark when a goal meets the measurability requirement and a zero (0) when the goal does not. Then revise each of the goals that does not meet all of the RUMBA requirements.

Goal	Relevant	Understandable	Measurable	Behavioral	Achievable
1. Arrive at work every day on time.					
2. Achieve the highest rating on most of my evaluations.					
3. Improve my ability to evaluate clients.					
4. By the end of next week, learn 5 new activities to use when working with stroke clients.					
5. Improve the accuracy of my documentation.					

The following is my revision of each goal so that it meets all of the RUMBA requirements:

1. ____

____

2. ____

____

3. ____

____

4. ____

____

5. ____

____

Writing Professional Goals

Write two professional goals that you want to achieve during fieldwork. In Columns 2 through 6, briefly describe how each goal meets each of the RUMBA requirements.

Professional Goal 1	Reasonable	Understand-able	Measurable	Behavioral	Achievable
Professional Goal 2	**Reasonable**	**Understand-able**	**Measurable**	**Behavioral**	**Achievable**

Compilation of Necessary Fieldwork Information: At-a-Glance Checklist

Item	Location of Item	Comments
Supplies (consumables)		
Equipment and storage		
Forms		
Policy and procedure manuals		
Instructions for equipment		
Library and location of resource materials		
Other necessary items or information		

Levels of Competence Related to Clinical Skills and Need for Supervision

Level	Distinction	Guiding Principle	Type of Supervision Needed	Date Achieved
Novice Can follow basic rules	No distinctions between rules and context in which the rules are applied	Basic rules and procedures	Close	
Advanced beginner Can assess and adapt to deviations from rules and procedures	Actions dictated by rules versus actions dictated by situation	Important aspects of a situation	Close	
Competent entry-level practitioner Can assess and adapt to important aspects of a situation	Actions dictated by situation versus actions dictated by general plan	General principles	Routine	
Proficient professional Can assess and adapt to deviations from plan	Actuals dictated by general plan versus actions dictated by intuition	Patterns and scenarios	General	
Expert Can assess and adapt to deviations from a pattern; can focus on critical factors	Actions and situations are synonymous	Holistic, integrated images and intuition	Minimal	Not achievable during fieldwork

Gathering Information on a Team Before Joining

Agency or site name:
Type of team (i.e., focus, disciplines, purpose):
Purpose of the team:
Team goals or priorities (i.e., how the team knows if its work is completed):
Members or disciplines represented on the team:
• What would be my responsibilities as a member of the team?
• What would I need to know to carry out my team responsibilities?
• Where could I get help if I needed it?
• What skills would I be bringing to the team?
• How could I demonstrate support of other team members?

• What else could I do to help the team produce results and achieve its goals?
• What would I be expected to prepare and bring to team meetings?
• What else would I need to do or prepare for work on this particular team?

Frames of Reference and Fieldwork Sites

Fieldwork or clinical site:	Frame(s) of reference:
Types of clients (i.e., diagnoses or reason for referral):	How this frame of reference is applied with clients:
What would be common goals for intervention related to this frame of reference in this particular setting?	What other influences does this frame of reference have in this particular setting?

Fundamental Elements of Documentation

- Client's full name and case number on each page of documentation
- Date and type of occupational therapy contact
- Identification of type of documentation, agency, and department name
- Occupational therapy signature with first name or initial, last name, and professional designation
- When applicable on notes or reports, signature of the recorder directly at the end of the note without space left between the body of the note and the signature
- Countersignature by an occupational therapist on documentation written by students or occupational therapy assistants when required by law or by the facility
- Acceptable terminology defined within the boundaries of the setting
- Abbreviation usage as acceptable within the boundaries of the setting
- When no facility requirements are listed, errors are corrected by drawing a single line through an error and initialing the correction; correction fluid or tape and erasures are not acceptable
- Adherence to professional standards of terminology used to document occupational therapy
- Disposal of records within law and agency requirements
- Compliance with confidentiality standards
- Compliance with legal and agency requirements of storage of records

Learning by Example: Well-Written Documentation

Ask your supervisor to provide examples of well-written documentation specific to the site where you are doing your fieldwork. Then analyze the way that content is presented. What you'll be doing here is similar to completing chart reviews, as is done in every health care facility.

• What makes the documentation easy to read and understand?
• How does the writer include important information without being too wordy?
• What type of information is included in each section of the documentation?

Documentation and Report Tracking Sheet

- A tracking sheet does not have to be fancy to be effective.
- Photocopy this page or design your own.
- When listing events, use colors to denote particular responsibilities.
- For your own record of completion and to give you a sense of what you have accomplished, cross out tasks that are done.

Date/Day	Client 1	Client 2	Client 3	Client 4	Client 5

Calendar

Tasks	Tasks

Day/Date	HOURLY APPOINTMENT SCHEDULE	Day/Date

6 AM	6 AM
7 AM	7 AM
8 AM	8 AM
9 AM	9 AM
10 AM	10 AM
11 AM	11 AM
12 PM	12 PM
1 PM	1 PM
2 PM	2 PM
3 PM	3 PM
4 PM	4 PM
5 PM	5 PM
6 PM	6 PM

Notes:

Calendar

Tasks	Tasks

Day/Date	HOURLY APPOINTMENT SCHEDULE	Day/Date
6 AM		6 AM
7 AM		7 AM
8 AM		8 AM
9 AM		9 AM
10 AM		10 AM
11 AM		11 AM
12 PM		12 PM
1 PM		1 PM
2 PM		2 PM
3 PM		3 PM
4 PM		4 PM
5 PM		5 PM
6 PM		6 PM

Notes:

Calendar

Tasks	Tasks

Day/Date	HOURLY APPOINTMENT SCHEDULE	Day/Date
6 AM		6 AM
7 AM		7 AM
8 AM		8 AM
9 AM		9 AM
10 AM		10 AM
11 AM		11 AM
12 PM		12 PM
1 PM		1 PM
2 PM		2 PM
3 PM		3 PM
4 PM		4 PM
5 PM		5 PM
6 PM		6 PM

Notes:

Calendar

Tasks	**Tasks**

Day/Date	HOURLY APPOINTMENT SCHEDULE	Day/Date
6 AM ____		6 AM ____
7 AM ____		7 AM ____
8 AM ____		8 AM ____
9 AM ____		9 AM ____
10 AM ____		10 AM ____
11 AM ____		11 AM ____
12 PM ____		12 PM ____
1 PM ____		1 PM ____
2 PM ____		2 PM ____
3 PM ____		3 PM ____
4 PM ____		4 PM ____
5 PM ____		5 PM ____
6 PM ____		6 PM ____

Notes:

Calendar

Tasks	Tasks

Day/Date	HOURLY APPOINTMENT SCHEDULE	Day/Date

6 AM	6 AM
7 AM	7 AM
8 AM	8 AM
9 AM	9 AM
10 AM	10 AM
11 AM	11 AM
12 PM	12 PM
1 PM	1 PM
2 PM	2 PM
3 PM	3 PM
4 PM	4 PM
5 PM	5 PM
6 PM	6 PM

Notes:

Calendar

Tasks	Tasks

Day/Date	HOURLY APPOINTMENT SCHEDULE	Day/Date

6 AM ______	6 AM ______
7 AM ______	7 AM ______
8 AM ______	8 AM ______
9 AM ______	9 AM ______
10 AM ______	10 AM ______
11 AM ______	11 AM ______
12 PM ______	12 PM ______
1 PM ______	1 PM ______
2 PM ______	2 PM ______
3 PM ______	3 PM ______
4 PM ______	4 PM ______
5 PM ______	5 PM ______
6 PM ______	6 PM ______

Notes:

Calendar

Tasks	Tasks

Day/Date	HOURLY APPOINTMENT SCHEDULE	Day/Date
6 AM		6 AM
7 AM		7 AM
8 AM		8 AM
9 AM		9 AM
10 AM		10 AM
11 AM		11 AM
12 PM		12 PM
1 PM		1 PM
2 PM		2 PM
3 PM		3 PM
4 PM		4 PM
5 PM		5 PM
6 PM		6 PM

Notes:

Calendar

Tasks	**Tasks**

Day/Date	**HOURLY APPOINTMENT SCHEDULE**	**Day/Date**

6 AM	6 AM
7 AM	7 AM
8 AM	8 AM
9 AM	9 AM
10 AM	10 AM
11 AM	11 AM
12 PM	12 PM
1 PM	1 PM
2 PM	2 PM
3 PM	3 PM
4 PM	4 PM
5 PM	5 PM
6 PM	6 PM

Notes:

Calendar

Tasks	Tasks

Day/Date	HOURLY APPOINTMENT SCHEDULE	Day/Date
6 AM		6 AM
7 AM		7 AM
8 AM		8 AM
9 AM		9 AM
10 AM		10 AM
11 AM		11 AM
12 PM		12 PM
1 PM		1 PM
2 PM		2 PM
3 PM		3 PM
4 PM		4 PM
5 PM		5 PM
6 PM		6 PM

Notes:

Calendar

Tasks	Tasks

Day/Date	HOURLY APPOINTMENT SCHEDULE	Day/Date
6 AM		6 AM
7 AM		7 AM
8 AM		8 AM
9 AM		9 AM
10 AM		10 AM
11 AM		11 AM
12 PM		12 PM
1 PM		1 PM
2 PM		2 PM
3 PM		3 PM
4 PM		4 PM
5 PM		5 PM
6 PM		6 PM

Notes:

Calendar

Tasks	Tasks

Day/Date	HOURLY APPOINTMENT SCHEDULE	Day/Date

6 AM	6 AM
7 AM	7 AM
8 AM	8 AM
9 AM	9 AM
10 AM	10 AM
11 AM	11 AM
12 PM	12 PM
1 PM	1 PM
2 PM	2 PM
3 PM	3 PM
4 PM	4 PM
5 PM	5 PM
6 PM	6 PM

Notes:

Calendar

Tasks	**Tasks**

Day/Date	**HOURLY APPOINTMENT SCHEDULE**	**Day/Date**

6 AM	6 AM
7 AM	7 AM
8 AM	8 AM
9 AM	9 AM
10 AM	10 AM
11 AM	11 AM
12 PM	12 PM
1 PM	1 PM
2 PM	2 PM
3 PM	3 PM
4 PM	4 PM
5 PM	5 PM
6 PM	6 PM

Notes:

Calendar

Tasks	Tasks

Day/Date	HOURLY APPOINTMENT SCHEDULE	Day/Date

6 AM	6 AM
7 AM	7 AM
8 AM	8 AM
9 AM	9 AM
10 AM	10 AM
11 AM	11 AM
12 PM	12 PM
1 PM	1 PM
2 PM	2 PM
3 PM	3 PM
4 PM	4 PM
5 PM	5 PM
6 PM	6 PM

Notes:

Calendar

Tasks	**Tasks**

Day/Date	**HOURLY APPOINTMENT SCHEDULE**	**Day/Date**
6 AM		6 AM
7 AM		7 AM
8 AM		8 AM
9 AM		9 AM
10 AM		10 AM
11 AM		11 AM
12 PM		12 PM
1 PM		1 PM
2 PM		2 PM
3 PM		3 PM
4 PM		4 PM
5 PM		5 PM
6 PM		6 PM

Notes:

Calendar

Tasks	Tasks

Day/Date	HOURLY APPOINTMENT SCHEDULE	Day/Date

6 AM	6 AM
7 AM	7 AM
8 AM	8 AM
9 AM	9 AM
10 AM	10 AM
11 AM	11 AM
12 PM	12 PM
1 PM	1 PM
2 PM	2 PM
3 PM	3 PM
4 PM	4 PM
5 PM	5 PM
6 PM	6 PM

Notes:

Calendar

Tasks	**Tasks**

Day/Date	**HOURLY APPOINTMENT SCHEDULE**	**Day/Date**

6 AM	6 AM
7 AM	7 AM
8 AM	8 AM
9 AM	9 AM
10 AM	10 AM
11 AM	11 AM
12 PM	12 PM
1 PM	1 PM
2 PM	2 PM
3 PM	3 PM
4 PM	4 PM
5 PM	5 PM
6 PM	6 PM

Notes:

Calendar

Tasks		Tasks
Day/Date	HOURLY APPOINTMENT SCHEDULE	Day/Date
6 AM		6 AM
7 AM		7 AM
8 AM		8 AM
9 AM		9 AM
10 AM		10 AM
11 AM		11 AM
12 PM		12 PM
1 PM		1 PM
2 PM		2 PM
3 PM		3 PM
4 PM		4 PM
5 PM		5 PM
6 PM		6 PM

Notes:

Calendar

Tasks	Tasks

Day/Date	HOURLY APPOINTMENT SCHEDULE	Day/Date

6 AM	6 AM
7 AM	7 AM
8 AM	8 AM
9 AM	9 AM
10 AM	10 AM
11 AM	11 AM
12 PM	12 PM
1 PM	1 PM
2 PM	2 PM
3 PM	3 PM
4 PM	4 PM
5 PM	5 PM
6 PM	6 PM

Notes:

Calendar

Tasks			Tasks
Day/Date	HOURLY APPOINTMENT SCHEDULE		Day/Date
6 AM		6 AM	
7 AM		7 AM	
8 AM		8 AM	
9 AM		9 AM	
10 AM		10 AM	
11 AM		11 AM	
12 PM		12 PM	
1 PM		1 PM	
2 PM		2 PM	
3 PM		3 PM	
4 PM		4 PM	
5 PM		5 PM	
6 PM		6 PM	

Notes:

Calendar

Tasks		**Tasks**
Day/Date	**HOURLY APPOINTMENT SCHEDULE**	**Day/Date**
6 AM		6 AM
7 AM		7 AM
8 AM		8 AM
9 AM		9 AM
10 AM		10 AM
11 AM		11 AM
12 PM		12 PM
1 PM		1 PM
2 PM		2 PM
3 PM		3 PM
4 PM		4 PM
5 PM		5 PM
6 PM		6 PM

Notes:

Calendar

Tasks	Tasks

Day/Date	HOURLY APPOINTMENT SCHEDULE	Day/Date
6 AM		6 AM
7 AM		7 AM
8 AM		8 AM
9 AM		9 AM
10 AM		10 AM
11 AM		11 AM
12 PM		12 PM
1 PM		1 PM
2 PM		2 PM
3 PM		3 PM
4 PM		4 PM
5 PM		5 PM
6 PM		6 PM

Notes:

Calendar

Tasks	**Tasks**

Day/Date	HOURLY APPOINTMENT SCHEDULE	Day/Date
6 AM ______		6 AM ______
7 AM ______		7 AM ______
8 AM ______		8 AM ______
9 AM ______		9 AM ______
10 AM ______		10 AM ______
11 AM ______		11 AM ______
12 PM ______		12 PM ______
1 PM ______		1 PM ______
2 PM ______		2 PM ______
3 PM ______		3 PM ______
4 PM ______		4 PM ______
5 PM ______		5 PM ______
6 PM ______		6 PM ______

Notes:

Calendar

Tasks	Tasks

Day/Date	HOURLY APPOINTMENT SCHEDULE	Day/Date

6 AM	6 AM
7 AM	7 AM
8 AM	8 AM
9 AM	9 AM
10 AM	10 AM
11 AM	11 AM
12 PM	12 PM
1 PM	1 PM
2 PM	2 PM
3 PM	3 PM
4 PM	4 PM
5 PM	5 PM
6 PM	6 PM

Notes:

Calendar

Tasks	**Tasks**

Day/Date	HOURLY APPOINTMENT SCHEDULE	Day/Date
6 AM		6 AM
7 AM		7 AM
8 AM		8 AM
9 AM		9 AM
10 AM		10 AM
11 AM		11 AM
12 PM		12 PM
1 PM		1 PM
2 PM		2 PM
3 PM		3 PM
4 PM		4 PM
5 PM		5 PM
6 PM		6 PM

Notes:

Calendar

Tasks	Tasks

Day/Date	HOURLY APPOINTMENT SCHEDULE	Day/Date

6 AM	6 AM
7 AM	7 AM
8 AM	8 AM
9 AM	9 AM
10 AM	10 AM
11 AM	11 AM
12 PM	12 PM
1 PM	1 PM
2 PM	2 PM
3 PM	3 PM
4 PM	4 PM
5 PM	5 PM
6 PM	6 PM

Notes:

Calendar

Tasks	**Tasks**

Day/Date	**HOURLY APPOINTMENT SCHEDULE**	**Day/Date**

6 AM	6 AM
7 AM	7 AM
8 AM	8 AM
9 AM	9 AM
10 AM	10 AM
11 AM	11 AM
12 PM	12 PM
1 PM	1 PM
2 PM	2 PM
3 PM	3 PM
4 PM	4 PM
5 PM	5 PM
6 PM	6 PM

Notes:

Calendar

Tasks	Tasks

Day/Date	HOURLY APPOINTMENT SCHEDULE	Day/Date

6 AM	6 AM
7 AM	7 AM
8 AM	8 AM
9 AM	9 AM
10 AM	10 AM
11 AM	11 AM
12 PM	12 PM
1 PM	1 PM
2 PM	2 PM
3 PM	3 PM
4 PM	4 PM
5 PM	5 PM
6 PM	6 PM

Notes:

Calendar

Tasks	**Tasks**

Day/Date	**HOURLY APPOINTMENT SCHEDULE**	**Day/Date**

6 AM	6 AM
7 AM	7 AM
8 AM	8 AM
9 AM	9 AM
10 AM	10 AM
11 AM	11 AM
12 PM	12 PM
1 PM	1 PM
2 PM	2 PM
3 PM	3 PM
4 PM	4 PM
5 PM	5 PM
6 PM	6 PM

Notes:

Calendar

Tasks	Tasks

Day/Date	HOURLY APPOINTMENT SCHEDULE	Day/Date
6 AM		6 AM
7 AM		7 AM
8 AM		8 AM
9 AM		9 AM
10 AM		10 AM
11 AM		11 AM
12 PM		12 PM
1 PM		1 PM
2 PM		2 PM
3 PM		3 PM
4 PM		4 PM
5 PM		5 PM
6 PM		6 PM

Notes:

Calendar

Tasks	**Tasks**

Day/Date	HOURLY APPOINTMENT SCHEDULE	Day/Date

6 AM	6 AM
7 AM	7 AM
8 AM	8 AM
9 AM	9 AM
10 AM	10 AM
11 AM	11 AM
12 PM	12 PM
1 PM	1 PM
2 PM	2 PM
3 PM	3 PM
4 PM	4 PM
5 PM	5 PM
6 PM	6 PM

Notes: